ISRAELI COOKBOOK

Table of Contents

Disclaimer

Copyright © 2021

All Rights Reserved.

No part of this book can be transmitted or reproduced in any form including print, electronic, photocopying, scanning, mechanical or recording without prior written permission from the author.

While the author has taken utmost efforts to ensure the accuracy of the written content, all readers are advised to follow information mentioned herein at their own risk. The author cannot be held responsible for any personal or commercial damage caused by information. All readers are encouraged to seek professional advice when needed.

Introduction

If you have travelled to Israel or have seen pictures of Israel's streets, you will see many vendors selling mouthwatering dishes. Israel is known for its street food, and every vendor serves different dishes, such as falafel, Shakshuka, hummus and more. It is easy to find something you like in Israel.

While Israelis believe family is most important, they also believe food is an integral part of their lives. If you see a group of Israelis gathered around, you can bet there is going to be a lot of food served. Whether they choose to eat at a local food joint or cook at home, most Israelis seem to talk about or eat food.

Academics and food critics still debate whether true Israeli cuisine exists or not. While this debate is ongoing, Israelis have been developing and enjoying delicious food. Israelis use their society and culture to develop these foods. This cuisine is an example of a melting pot. Jews hail from many countries and have travelled across the globe, before they returned to Israel, their ancient land. They brought different recipes and foods they came across during their travels. These new recipes mingled with other dietary laws, rules and native ingredients Jews use.

Any cuisine is a result of a combination of different forces, such as agricultural, historical, and sociological. The same can be said for Israeli cuisine, as well. It is for this reason many foods considered to be an integral part of the Israeli cuisine originated from different cuisines in the Middle East, including the famous salad of tomatoes and cucumbers or falafel. Israeli cuisine is also influenced by Eastern European Jewish traditions. Therefore, you may find some recipes with sour cream and borscht.

It should come as no surprise that Israeli cuisine is influenced by geography. Therefore, different foods, such as olive oil, olives, yogurt, chickpeas, and wheat are an important part of the cuisine. Some dietary laws also have an influence on Israeli cuisine, including aversions to shellfish, pork and other foods and separating meat and milk. Additionally, Jewish festivals and holidays have also shaped Israeli cuisine.

Israelis also believe lunch is their focal meal of the day and not dinner, like the people living in the Mediterranean region. While the debate over where most Israeli foods originated from is ongoing, you may hear a different story from the locals. The truth is there is no evidence to determine when foods, such as shawarma, falafel, hummus, Kanafeh and Shakshuka became popular in Israel. Unfortunately, no evidence exists to determine when these foods became a part of the Israeli cuisine, but every side of the border claims the food is theirs.

Hummus is a staple food in every home and falafel is a favorite fast food for all Israelis. Israelis also love eating eggs because it is an important protein source. Israelis also cook vegetables and fruit in different ways, making them taste wonderful. They cook them in creative ways. Some Israelis eat vegetables for breakfast because they prefer starting their day off in a healthy way.

Despite the controversy surrounding Israeli food, one thing most people agree on is that the food is creative and delicious. If you want to learn how to cook different foods, you have come to the right place. This book has some of the best Israeli recipes. The instructions are easy to follow, and the ingredients can be found easily in the supermarket near your house. You can tweak these recipes in case you do not find some ingredients and create your own recipes.

Thank you for purchasing the book. I hope you and your family enjoy the delicious recipes in this book.

Chapter One: Breakfast recipes

Israeli Pita Bread (Pitot)

Preparation time: About 2 hours

Cooking time: 6 minutes

Number of servings: 4

Ingredients:

- 1 ¼ teaspoons active dry yeast
- ½ teaspoon granulated sugar
- 2 cups unbleached all-purpose flour
- ½ cup + 1/3 cup warm water (95° F)
- ½ teaspoon sea salt

Directions:

1. You can make the dough in a stand mixer or use your hands to do so.
2. I am using the stand mixer. Add warm water, sugar, and yeast into the mixing bowl of the stand mixer. Stir and set aside for 5 – 10 minutes until a little frothy. If the mixture doesn't become frothy, discard the mixture and make a fresh mixture.
3. Fix the stand mixer with dough hook attachment.
4. Add flour and salt into another bowl and stir. Set the mixer on low speed.

5. Add about a cup of the flour mixture into the mixing bowl and mix until well incorporated.
6. Add the remaining flour and mix until dough is formed. The dough will be sticky.
7. Remove the dough hook attachment.
8. Cover the bowl with cling wrap and place in a warm place until it doubles in size. It may take an hour.
9. Place a sheet of parchment paper on a large baking sheet. Dust parchment paper with some flour.
10. Dust your hands generously with flour. Divide the dough into 4 equal portions and shape into balls. Place the balls on the baking sheet. Sprinkle some flour on top of the dough and cover it loosely with plastic wrap.
11. Let it rest for about 10 minutes.
12. Place the rack 8 inches below the top-heating element in the oven.
13. Place a pizza stone in the oven and preheat the oven to 500° F.
14. Dust your countertop with some flour.
15. Dust your hands once again and take a ball of dough. Place it on your countertop. Dust the rolling pin with flour as well. Roll it with your hands into a pita of about 6 inches diameter and place on the baking sheet.
16. Repeat with the remaining balls of dough, dusting your hands with flour each time. Leave some gap between each of the pita rounds on the baking sheet.
17. Open the oven and quickly place 2 of the rolled pita on the pizza stone. Make sure the pitas lie flat.

18. Bake for about 5 – 7 minutes. Watch them after about 5 minutes of baking as they can get burnt.
19. Remove the pitas from the oven and place on a plate.
20. Bake the remaining pitas similarly.
21. If you do not have a pizza stone, you can keep a baking sheet while preheating the oven.
22. You can serve it with hummus, falafel, shawarma, and baba ganoush, Shakshuka etc. You can also fill some salad in the pitas and serve.

Classic Shakshuka

Preparation time: 10 minutes

Cooking time: 15 – 18 minutes

Number of servings: 4

Ingredients:

- ½ onion, chopped
- ½ yellow bell pepper, diced
- 1 clove garlic, sliced
- ¼ teaspoon sugar (optional)
- 2 eggs
- 1 ½ tablespoons olive oil
- ¼ teaspoon ground cumin
- Salt to taste
- ½ teaspoon sweet paprika
- Freshly ground pepper to taste
- ½ ripe tomato, chopped
- ½ cup canned chopped tomatoes
- ¼ teaspoon cayenne pepper flakes or thinly sliced red chili pepper
- ¼ cup water or as required
- Chopped fresh cilantro or parsley, to garnish

Directions:

1. Place a heavy bottomed skillet over medium heat. Add oil and allow it to heat.
2. Add onion and cook for a couple of minutes. Add bell pepper and cook until onions are tender.
3. Stir in the garlic and cook for a couple of minutes until aromatic.
4. Stir in the tomatoes (fresh and canned), salt, cumin, pepper, cayenne pepper, and sugar. Add a little water and stir. Cover and cook for about 15 minutes. Stir occasionally. The gravy should not be watery. Cook until thick.
5. Make 2 cavities at different spots, in the mixture. Crack an egg into each cavity. Cover and cook until the eggs are cooked as per your preference.
6. Sprinkle parsley on top. Season the eggs with salt and pepper.
7. This can be served with pita bread or flatbread.

Green Shakshuka

Preparation time: 10 minutes

Cooking time: 30 minutes

Number of servings: 3

Ingredients:

- ½ onion
- 3 cups mixed greens (like kale, spinach, Collard greens, Swiss chard etc.), thinly sliced
- ¼ cup yogurt or sour cream
- 2 small cloves garlic, sliced
- ¼ fresh jalapeño, deseeded, sliced
- A wee bit ground nutmeg
- Pepper to taste
- 1.8 ounces feta cheese or fresh goat cheese
- Salt to taste
- 3 eggs
- 1 teaspoon oil

Directions:

1. Place a heavy bottomed skillet over medium heat. Add oil and allow it to heat.
2. Add onion and cook for a couple of minutes, until translucent.

3. Stir in the garlic and cook for about a minute until aromatic.
4. Stir in the mixed greens. Cover and cook for about 10 minutes on low heat until the greens wilt. Stir occasionally.
5. Stir in salt, pepper, nutmeg, and yogurt.
6. Make 3 cavities at different spots, in the mixture. Crack an egg into each cavity. Cover and cook until the eggs are cooked as per your preference.
7. Sprinkle feta cheese on top. Season the eggs with salt and pepper.
8. This can be served with pita bread or flatbread.

Cheese Bourekas

Preparation time: 15 minutes

Cooking time: 20 minutes

Number of servings: 24

Ingredients:

- 2 eggs, lightly beaten
- 2 large eggs, beaten, for egg wash
- 2 teaspoons dried parsley
- 1 teaspoon garlic salt
- ½ teaspoon onion powder
- ½ teaspoon pepper
- 2 packages frozen (17.5 ounces each) puff pastry
- Sesame seeds to garnish
- 16 ounces shredded mozzarella cheese
- Little water to moisten

Directions:

1. Set the temperature of the oven to 350° F and preheat the oven.
2. Add cheese, parsley, onion powder, garlic powder, and salt into the bowl of beaten egg and whisk well.
3. Dust your countertop with some flour.

4. Place the puff pastry sheets on the countertop and cut into 5 inch square pieces.
5. Brush lightly the edges of all the squares with a little water.
6. Divide the cheese filling among the squares and place on the squares towards one of the corners. You should be placing about a heaping tablespoon of filling on each square. Fold each in half, diagonally (the opposite end). So you get triangular shaped bourekas.
7. Press the edges to seal. You can use a fork for sealing.
8. Place the bourekas on a greased baking sheet. Brush the top of bourekas with egg wash.
9. Scatter sesame seeds on top.
10. Place the baking sheet in the oven and bake until golden brown.
11. Remove from the oven and cool for 5 minutes.
12. Serve.

Semolina Porridge

Preparation time: 5 minutes

Cooking time: 15 minutes

Number of servings: 4 – 5

Ingredients:

- 4 cups milk of your choice
- 2/3 cup semolina
- 1/8 teaspoon salt
- 2 cups water
- 2 tablespoons sugar
- Cinnamon to garnish (optional)

Directions:

1. Combine milk and water in a saucepan and place the saucepan over medium heat.
2. When the mixture starts boiling, lower the heat and pour in the semolina, stirring constantly while adding.
3. Stir in sugar and salt and cook until thick and porridge-like. Stir frequently.
4. Serve in bowls. Garnish with cinnamon if using and serve.

Classic Potato Latkes (Israeli Potato Pancakes)

Preparation time: 30 minutes

Cooking time: 30 minutes

Number of servings: 12

Ingredients:

- 1 ¼ pounds potatoes, peeled, rinsed
- 6 tablespoons matzo meal or breadcrumbs
- ½ tablespoon potato starch or more if required
- ¼ teaspoon pepper
- ½ large onion, shredded
- 1 large egg, beaten
- ¾ teaspoon salt or to taste
- 1/8 cup schmaltz
- Oil of deep frying like avocado oil or peanut oil or any high smoking oils

Directions:

1. Grate the potatoes with a hand grater or in the food processor. Immerse the grated potatoes into a bowl of cold water. Drain off in a colander after a minute or so.
2. Place a cooling rack on a baking sheet next to your stovetop.

3. Take 2 layers of cheesecloth and place potato and onion in the center. Bring the edges of the cheesecloth together and squeeze out as much moisture as possible from the potatoes. Place the potatoes in a bowl.
4. Pour enough oil into a skillet such that it is about 1/8 inch in height from the bottom of the pan. Add schmaltz if using, into the skillet. Let the oil heat.
5. Meanwhile, add egg, potato starch, matzo meal, pepper, and salt into the bowl of potatoes and stir using a fork until well combined.
6. When the oil is hot, take about 3 tablespoons of the mixture and shape into a patty and place it in the pan. Make another 2 – 3 of the latkes and place in the skillet.
7. When the underside is golden brown, turn the latkes over and cook the other side until golden brown.
8. Remove with a slotted spoon and place on the rack.
9. Make the remaining latkes and cook them in a similar manner.

Sabich

Preparation time: 30 minutes

Cooking time: 40 minutes

Number of servings: 8

Ingredients:

- Extra-virgin olive oil, as required
- 2 seedless cucumber, peeled, diced
- 2 pint grape tomatoes, diced
- 4 tablespoons fresh lemon juice
- 1 tablespoon grated lemon zest
- 4 – 5 tablespoons minced, flat-leaf parsley
- 4 tablespoons white wine vinegar
- Kosher salt to taste
- 2 large eggplants, cut into ½ inch thick round slices
- 2 large cloves garlic, grated
- ½ head cabbage, thinly shredded (about 2 cups)
- 2/3 cup tahini

To serve:

- 8 hard-boiled eggs, peeled, sliced
- Amba, as required
- Israeli pickles, as required

- 8 fresh round pita bread, warmed, split slightly to make a pocket

Directions:

1. Set the temperature of the oven to 375° F and preheat the oven.
2. Prepare a baking sheet by lining it with parchment paper.
3. Add tomatoes, cucumber, parsley, about 2 tablespoons oil, and lemon juice into a bowl and toss well, add a pinch of salt and pepper and toss well. Cover and set it aside for a while for the flavors to meld.
4. Place eggplant slices on the baking sheet. Drizzle oil over the eggplant slices. Sprinkle salt and pepper.
5. Place the baking sheet in the oven and bake until the slices are brown. Flip sides after 15 minutes of baking, about 25 – 30 minutes.
6. Place cabbage in a bowl. Add vinegar and a little salt and toss well.
7. Meanwhile, whisk together tahini, salt, garlic, lemon juice, and lemon zest in a bowl. Keep whisking until the color turns a little pale.
8. Add about ½ cup of the tahini sauce into the bowl of cabbage and mix well.
9. Spread a little of the tahini sauce inside each pita pocket. Place a few eggplant slices inside each pita pocket. Stuff some of the cabbage in the pockets. Place egg slices and Israeli pickles. Spoon some more tahini sauce if remaining.

10. Next stuff some tomato salad in each pita. Finally spoon amba and serve right away.

Israeli Breakfast Salad

Preparation time: 10 minutes

Cooking time: 0 minutes

Number of servings: 2

Ingredients:

- 1 medium cucumber, peeled, halved lengthwise
- ¼ cup crumbled feta cheese
- ½ green bell pepper, deseeded, finely chopped
- Salt to taste
- Black pepper to taste
- 2 tablespoons olive oil
- ¼ cup cottage cheese
- 2 tablespoons grated onion, drained
- 2 tablespoons fresh lemon juice
- Fresh mint sprigs to garnish

Directions:

1. Prick the cucumber with a fork all over and season with salt. Place it in a strainer for 30 minutes. Chop the cucumber into smaller pieces and add into a bowl.
2. Add feta cheese, bell pepper, salt, pepper, oil, cottage cheese, onion, and lemon juice and stir well.
3. Garnish with mint sprigs.

4. Cover and Set aside for 30 minutes for the flavors to infuse
    before serving.

Tahini Date Shake

Preparation time: 5 minutes + freezing time

Cooking time: 0 minutes

Number of servings: 2

Ingredients:

- 1 cup milk of your choice
- 4 tablespoons tahini paste
- ¼ teaspoon vanilla extract
- 2 ripe banana, peeled, sliced
- 5 medjool dates, pitted, chopped
- ½ teaspoon ground cinnamon or to taste
- Ice cubes, as required

Directions:

1. Place banana slices on a tray and freeze until firm (about 1 ½ - 2 hours).
2. Add milk, tahini, vanilla, banana, dates, and cinnamon into a blender.
3. Blend until smooth.
4. Add into 2 glasses and serve.

Labneh (Yogurt Cheese)

Preparation time: 8 hours

Cooking time: 0 minutes

Number of servings: 4 – 6 (makes about 2 cups)

Ingredients:

- 16 ounces Greek or plain yogurt (Greek yogurt is recommended)
- 1 cup extra-virgin olive oil
- ½ tablespoon minced, fresh herbs (like mint, thyme, chives or parsley)
- Salt to taste
- Za'atar to sprinkle

Directions:

1. Combine salt and yogurt in a bowl.
2. Place yogurt on a double-layered cheesecloth. Place the cheesecloth along with yogurt on a wire mesh strainer placed over a bowl.
3. Shift this entire setup into the refrigerator and let it drain for 8 – 9 hours. The collected whey can be discarded or used in some other recipe like a smoothie.

4. Remove the cheesecloth and transfer the cheese into a jar. Add seasonings and herbs and stir well. Drizzle oil over it. Sprinkle za'atar seasoning on top.
5. Close the lid of the jar. Refrigerate until use. It can last for a week.
6. The collected liquid is called whey and can be used in some other recipe like a smoothie or pickles etc.

Chapter Two: Shawarma Recipes

Shawarma Spice Mix

Preparation time: 5 minutes

Cooking time: 3 – 4 minutes if using whole spices

Makes: About 2/3 cup

Ingredients:

<u>Using powdered spices:</u>

- 4 teaspoons ground cumin
- 4 teaspoons ground cinnamon
- 2 teaspoons ground nutmeg
- 2 teaspoons cayenne pepper powder or hot paprika
- 1 teaspoon ground cloves
- 2 teaspoons ground allspice
- 4 teaspoons garlic powder
- 2 teaspoons ground cardamom
- 4 teaspoons sweet paprika
- 1 teaspoon turmeric powder
- 2 teaspoons ginger powder
- 2 teaspoons ground black pepper

<u>If using whole spices:</u>

- 2 teaspoons cumin seeds
- 2 inches stick cinnamon

- ½ inch whole nutmeg
- 4 whole dried cayenne peppers or paprika
- 10 whole cloves
- 10 allspice berries
- 4 teaspoons garlic powder
- 10 cardamom pods
- 6 dry whole paprika
- 1 teaspoon turmeric powder
- 2 teaspoons ginger powder
- 20 black peppercorns

Directions:

1. To make shawarma powder using powdered spices: Place all the powdered spices in a bowl and mix really well using a spoon until well combined.
2. Spoon into an airtight container and close the lid. Place in a cool and dark area. It can last for 3 – 4 months.
3. To make shawarma powder using whole spices: Combine all the whole spices in a pan.
4. Place the pan over low heat and let it heat for about 3 – 4 minutes, stirring occasionally until fragrant.
5. Turn off the heat and let it cool to room temperature.
6. Transfer the whole spices into a spice grinder. Also add powdered spices and blend until finely powdered.
7. Spoon into an airtight container and close the lid. Place in a cool and dark area. It can last for 3 – 4 months.

Tahini Sauce

Preparation time: 5 minutes

Cooking time: 0 minutes

Makes: About 2/3 cup

Ingredients:

- 4 cloves garlic, minced
- Salt to taste
- ½ cup tahini paste
- ¾ cup lemon juice
- 6 – 8 tablespoons water

Directions:

1. Place garlic and salt in a bowl. Mash together the garlic and salt until a paste is made. Add tahini paste, lemon juice, and water. Whisk well. You can also blend the ingredients in a blender until smooth.
2. Refrigerate until use. Consume within 5 days.

Tzatziki

Preparation time: 1 hour and 20 minutes

Cooking time: 0 minutes

Makes: About 1 ¼ cups

Ingredients:

- 5 ounces cucumber, peeled, halved, deseeded, grated
- ½ tablespoon chopped fresh dill leaves
- ¾ tablespoon white vinegar
- 1/8 teaspoon kosher salt
- ½ clove garlic, minced
- 9 ounces full-fat Greek yogurt
- ½ tablespoon olive oil + extra to drizzle if desired
- Freshly ground pepper to taste
- ¾ tablespoon white wine vinegar
- Dill sprig to garnish (optional)

Directions:

1. Squeeze out as much liquid as possible from the cucumber.
2. Place the squeezed cucumber in a strainer and place the strainer over a bowl.
3. Add salt and mix well. Let it rest for 10 – 15 minutes.

4. Once again squeeze out as much liquid as possible from the cucumber.
5. Combine cucumber, dill, Greek yogurt, oil, pepper, salt, and garlic in a bowl.
6. Cover the bowl and place it in the refrigerator for about an hour.
7. Trickle some oil on top if desired.

Chicken Shawarma

Preparation time: 10 minutes

Cooking time: 20 minutes

Number of servings: 8

Ingredients:

- ¼ cup finely chopped fresh parsley
- 2 teaspoons shawarma spice blend
- ¼ teaspoon coriander powder
- 1 teaspoon salt
- 4 tablespoons fresh lemon juice, divided
- 2 pounds chicken breast halves, skinless, boneless, thinly sliced
- 2 tablespoons tahini
- 10 tablespoons plain low--fat Greek-style yogurt, divided
- 2 garlic cloves, minced
- ¼ cup extra-virgin olive oil

To serve:

- 8 (6-inch each) pitas, halved
- 1 cup chopped plum tomatoes
- 1 cup chopped cucumber
- ½ cup chopped red onion

35

Directions:

1. Add salt, shawarma spice, parsley, 2 tablespoons yogurt, and 2 tablespoons lemon juice into a large bowl. Mix well.
2. Add chicken into the bowl. Stir to coat the chicken well.
3. Place a large nonstick skillet over medium heat. Add oil. When the oil is hot, add chicken into the skillet and cook the chicken until brown all over and cooked through as well. Stir often. Cook in batches if required.
4. Meanwhile, add the remaining yogurt, and lemon juice into a bowl. Add tahini and garlic and mix well. Smear the yogurt mixture inside the pita bread halves. Divide equally the chicken, cucumber, tomatoes, and onions among the pita halves.
5. Serve.

Beef Shawarma

Preparation time: 20 minutes

Cooking time: 10 minutes

Number of servings: 4

Ingredients:

- 2 ½ teaspoons shawarma spice blend
- 2 tablespoons extra-virgin olive
- Juice of ½ lemon

- Kosher salt to taste
- ½ medium onion, sliced
- Pepper to taste
- 2 tablespoons white wine vinegar
- ¾ pound beef flap steak or flank steak, 2 cloves garlic, minced

To serve:

- 2 (6-inch each) pitas, halved
- ¼ cup chopped plum tomatoes
- ¼ cup chopped cucumber
- ¼ cup chopped red onion
- Tahini sauce
- Pickled cucumbers

Directions:

1. Combine shawarma spice blend, oil, vinegar, lemon juice, and lemon zest in a bowl.
2. Thinly slice the steak against the grain into bite size pieces and add into the bowl of spice blend mixture. Also add onion and garlic and mix well.
3. Cover and set aside for 15 minutes. If you have time on hand, you can place it in the refrigerator for a few hours to marinate.
4. Place a skillet or cast-iron pan over high heat. Add meat and onions into the pan and cook the meat. In 10 – 15 minutes the meat will be cooked.

5. Smear the tahini sauce inside the pita bread halves. Divide equally the water, cucumber, tomatoes, and onions among the pita halves. Place some pickled cucumbers in the pita halves and serve.

Cauliflower Shawarma

Preparation time: minutes

Cooking time: minutes

Number of servings: 6

Ingredients:

- 2 small heads cauliflower, cut into florets
- 1 teaspoon salt or to taste
- 1 teaspoon cayenne or to taste
- ½ cup water
- 4 teaspoons oil
- 2 teaspoons garlic paste or 1 teaspoon garlic granules
- 4 – 6 teaspoons shawarma spice blend or to taste

To serve:

- 6 pita bread or yeast-free flatbreads, warmed
- 1 cup chopped plum tomatoes
- 1 cup chopped cucumber or cucumber pickles
- ½ cup chopped red onion
- Lettuce leaves as required, chopped

- Tahini sauce, as required
- Hummus, as required
- A handful fresh cilantro, chopped

Directions:

1. Place a large skillet over medium heat and cauliflower, water, and salt. Cook covered until tender.
2. Add spice blend, oil, garlic, salt, and cayenne into a bowl and stir. Pour this mixture over the cauliflower and toss well.
3. Cook for 2-3 minutes until fragrant. Taste and adjust the seasonings and salt if necessary.
4. Spread a generous amount of hummus over the pita or flatbread or cut into 2 halves and spread it inside the pita pockets. Place cauliflower, tomatoes, cucumber, and lettuce.
5. Spoon some tahini sauce. Sprinkle cilantro and serve.

Israeli Vegan Shawarma

Preparation time: 30 minutes

Cooking time: 60 minutes

Number of servings: 6

Ingredients:

- 3.5 ounces dried Yuba wings
- 7 ounces king oyster mushrooms, thinly sliced
- 6 – 10 cloves garlic, peeled, sliced
- 6 tablespoons shawarma spice blend
- 1 teaspoon salt or to taste
- 7 ounces tofu
- 2 onions, halved, thinly sliced
- 2/3 cup olive oil
- 2 teaspoons paprika

To serve:

- 6 pita bread
- Amba sauce
- Fried eggplant
- Fries
- Tahini sauce
- Hummus
- 1 cup chopped plum tomatoes

- 1 cup chopped cucumber
- ½ cup chopped red onion
- Chopped parsley

Directions:

1. Set the temperature of the oven to 390° F and preheat the oven. Prepare a baking dish by lining it with parchment paper
2. Pour boiling water over the Yuba wings in a bowl. Let it rehydrate for 5 minutes. Drain and rinse well. Squeeze out as much moisture as possible from the Yuba wings. Once done with the squeezing, cut it on the side and keep it in the baking dish.
3. Place tofu, onion, mushrooms and garlic in the baking dish. Sprinkle shawarma spice blend, salt, and paprika on top. Drizzle oil and stir until well combined. Spread the mixture all over the pan.
4. Bake for about 30 minutes, stirring the mixture after 15 minutes of baking. Bake until crisp and brown.
5. Cut off a thin slice from the top of each pita to make pockets. Apply hummus on the inner sides of the pita pockets.
6. Divide the shawarma among the pockets. Fill it up with fries, and fried eggplant. Place tomatoes, cucumber, and onion. Drizzle amba sauce and tahini in the pockets. Sprinkle parsley and serve.

Lamb Shawarma

Preparation time: 8 – 9 hours

Cooking time: 3 – 4 hours

Number of servings: 4

Ingredients:

- 3 tablespoons shawarma spice blend or more to taste
- ½ tablespoon sumac
- 1 ½ inches fresh ginger, peeled, grated
- 1/3 cup chopped cilantro
- ¼ cup neutral oil of your choice
- ½ teaspoon kosher salt or to taste
- 2 cloves garlic, peeled, crushed
- 2 tablespoons fresh lemon juice
- 1 leg of lamb, bone-in, about 3 – 4 pounds

Directions:

1. To make marinade: Combine shawarma spice blend, sumac, ginger, cilantro, oil, salt, garlic, and lemon juice in a bowl.
2. Make slits on the meat at 5 – 6 places using a knife. The slits should be about ½ inch deep. Keep it in a roasting pan.

3. Spread the marinade all over the meat and rub it well into it. Place the meat with the fat side on top and keep the pan covered with foil. Let it marinate at room temperature for 2 – 3 hours or in the refrigerator for 8 – 9 hours (placing in the refrigerator is recommended)
4. Set the temperature of the oven to 350° F and preheat the oven. Uncover the meat and place the roasting pan in the oven.
5. Cook for about 3 – 4 hours or until the meat is cooked.
6. Once the meat has cooked for about 30 minutes, pour a cup of boiling water into the roasting pan.
7. Baste the meat with this water from the pan every 40 – 50 minutes. When the meat has cooked for about 1-½ hours, cover the meat once again with foil and roast for the remaining time, until meat is cooked.
8. Remove meat from the oven and place on your cutting board. Let it rest for 10 – 15 minutes.
9. Slice and serve.

Chickpea Shawarma

Preparation time: 5 minutes

Cooking time: 30 minutes

Number of servings: 8

Ingredients:

For chickpeas:

- 2 cans (15 ounces each) chickpeas, rinsed, drained, dried with paper towels
- 2 – 3 tablespoons shawarma spice blend
- 2 tablespoons grapeseed or avocado oil
- 1 teaspoon sea salt

For garlic dill sauce:

- ½ cup hummus or tahini
- 2 teaspoons dried dill
- 4 – 6 tablespoons water or almond milk
- 2 tablespoons lemon juice
- 6 cloves garlic, minced
- Sea salt to taste

To serve:

- Pita or flatbread, warmed
- Onion slices (optional
- Tomato slices and Chili garlic sauce (optional)
- Romaine lettuce leaves or parsley, chopped (optional)

Directions:

1. Set the temperature of the oven to 425° F and preheat the oven. Prepare 2 large baking sheets with parchment paper.
2. Spread chickpeas on a clean kitchen towel. Take some paper towels and dry the chickpeas. Dry them as much as possible. Add chickpeas into a bowl. Drizzle oil over it and toss. In a bowl. Sprinkle shawarma spice blend over it and toss well. Transfer onto the prepared baking sheets. Spread it evenly, in a single layer, without overlapping.
3. Place the baking sheets on 2 racks in the oven. Bake crisp and golden brown in color. Make sure to stir the chickpeas after about 15 minutes of baking and interchange the baking sheets on the rack.
4. When done, cool the chickpeas for a while. Taste and adjust the seasonings if required.
5. For garlic dill sauce: Meanwhile, add all the ingredients for garlic dill sauce into a bowl and stir until well combined. Cover and set aside for a while for the flavors to meld.
6. To serve: Cut off a thin slice from one of the edges of the pita bread to make pocket. Fill the pita pockets with chickpeas among the pitas. Fill the pockets with onion, tomato, and lettuce leaves if using. Drizzle garlic dill sauce and chili garlic sauce if using.

7. Leftover chickpeas and sauce can be placed in separate airtight containers in the refrigerator for 3 to 4 days. You can also use the chickpeas as a snack.

Veggie Shawarma Bowls

Preparation time: 15 minutes

Cooking time: 25 - 35 minutes

Number of servings: 8

Ingredients:

- 2 cans (15 ounces each) chickpeas, drained, rinsed
- 2 sweet potatoes, peeled, cut into ½ inch cubes
- 2 small heads cauliflower, cut into bite size florets
- 2 teaspoon kosher salt or to taste
- Juice of a lemon
- Pepper to taste
- 2 – 4 teaspoons shawarma spice blend or more to taste

For the bowls

- Cooked quinoa
- 1 cup chopped plum tomatoes
- 1 cup chopped cucumber or cucumber pickles
- ½ cup chopped red onion
- Lettuce leaves or cabbage as required, thinly sliced
- Tahini sauce, as required
- A handful fresh cilantro or parsley, chopped
- Feta cheese, crumbled

Directions:

1. Set the temperature of the oven to 425° F and preheat the oven. Prepare 2 large baking sheets with parchment paper.
2. Spread chickpeas on a clean kitchen towel. Take some paper towels and dry the chickpeas. Dry them as much as possible.
3. Combine chickpeas, cauliflower, and sweet potatoes in a bowl. Add salt, pepper, and shawarma spice blend and toss well. Spread the mixture on baking sheets.
4. Place both the baking sheets in the oven and bake until vegetables and chickpeas are cooked and brown. Stir the mixture half way through roasting.
5. Interchange the baking sheets on the oven racks.
6. Take out the baking sheets from the oven and sprinkle lemon juice.
7. Place cooked quinoa in serving bowls. Place the roasted vegetable mixture over the quinoa. Place lettuce, cucumber, red onion, tomato, and feta over the vegetable mixture, in layers.
8. Drizzle tahini sauce on top and serve.

The end… almost!

<u>A Short message from the Author:</u>

Hey, are you enjoying the book? I'd love to hear your thoughts!

Many readers do not know how hard reviews are to come by, and how much they help an author.

I would be incredibly thankful if you could take just 60 seconds to write a brief review on Amazon, even if it's just a few sentences!

Please head to the product page, and leave a review as shown below.

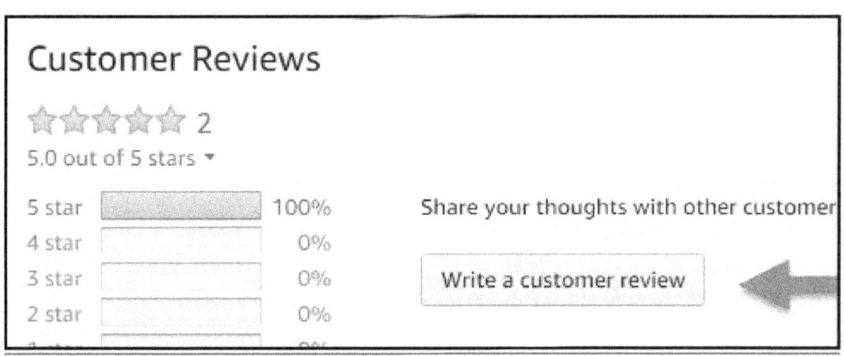

Thank you for taking the time to share your thoughts!

Chapter Three: Hummus Recipes

Hummus

Preparation time: 8 – 9 hours

Cooking time: 50 – 60 minutes

Makes: About 1 ½ cups

Ingredients:

- ½ cup dried chickpeas
- ½ tablespoon + ½ teaspoon sea salt, divided
- 2 – 3 cloves garlic, peeled
- 2 tablespoons lemon juice
- ¼ teaspoon ground cumin
- 1 teaspoon baking soda, divided
- 2 small bay leaves
- ¼ whole onion
- 1/3 cup tahini
- ½ cup cooked chickpea water
- Extra salt to taste

<u>To garnish:</u>

- Extra-virgin olive oil
- Chopped parsley
- Chopped kalamata olives

Directions:

1. Rinse chickpeas well and place in a bowl. Pour enough water into the bowl such that the chickpeas are covered with at least 3 inches of water (about 2 – 3 cups water)
2. Add ½ tablespoon sea salt and ½ teaspoon baking soda. Place the bowl in the refrigerator overnight, 8 – 9 hours.
3. The following morning, drain off the water and rinse well. If you have a pressure cooker or instant pot, cook it in it, it is quicker. If you do not have a pressure cooker, cook it in a saucepan.
4. Cook the chickpeas by the chosen method. Combine chickpeas, ½ teaspoon baking soda, ½ teaspoon salt, bay leaves, onion, and a clove of garlic in the pressure cooker or saucepan and pour enough water to cover the chickpeas by 2 inches in height, above the chickpeas.
5. Cook on High for 10 minutes and let the pressure release naturally. Whatever is your method of cooking, make sure to cook the chickpeas until soft.
6. Meanwhile, mince the remaining cloves of garlic and mash it up well into a paste in a bowl.
7. Add lemon juice and a pinch of salt to the bowl containing garlic. Stir and keep it aside.
8. Drain the chickpeas into a strainer placed over a bowl. The cooked liquid is to be retained.
9. Discard the onion and bay leaves.
10. Place tahini in a blender or food processor. Add about a tablespoon of water and blend. Keep adding a tablespoon

of water and blending, until you get smooth and free flowing tahini.

11. Add chickpeas along with the cooked garlic and cumin into the blender and blend until smooth, adding 2 – 3 tablespoons of cooked water while blending. You can add more water if desired.

12. Transfer the hummus into a serving bowl.

13. Drizzle some olive oil over the hummus. Garnish with parsley and olives.

14. Keep the bowl covered in the refrigerator until ready to serve.

Black-Eyed Pea Hummus

Preparation time: 5 minutes

Cooking time: 3 – 4 minutes if using whole spices

Makes: About 1 ¾ cups

Ingredients:

- 1 – 2 cloves garlic, peeled, minced
- 3 tablespoons tahini
- ¼ teaspoon salt or to taste
- 1 can (from a 15.5 ounces can) black-eyed peas, drained
- ¼ cup fresh lemon juice
- ½ teaspoon ground cumin
- ¼ teaspoon paprika
- Chopped chives to garnish (optional)

Directions:

1. Place garlic, lemon juice, tahini, salt, black-eyed peas, cumin, and paprika in the food processor bowl and process until smooth.
2. Transfer into a bowl. Sprinkle chives on top. Keep the bowl covered in the refrigerator until ready to serve.

Fava Bean Hummus

Preparation time: 3 – 4 hours

Cooking time: 30 – 40 minutes

Makes: About 2 cups

Ingredients:

- ½ cup cooked chickpeas
- 1 cup uncooked dried fava beans, rinsed well
- ½ tablespoon lemon juice
- 1 clove garlic, peeled
- ½ teaspoon dried thyme
- ½ teaspoon dried oregano
- 3 teaspoons tahini
- Salt to taste

<u>To garnish:</u>

- Black sesame seeds
- Minced garlic
- Chopped fresh thyme

Directions:

1. Soak fava beans in water. The water should be at least 3 inches above the beans. Let it soak for 3 – 4 hours.
2. Drain off the water. If you have a pressure cooker or instant pot, cook it in it, it is quicker. If you do not have a pressure cooker, cook it in a saucepan.
3. Cook the fava beans by the chosen method. Cook until soft. It should take about 25 – 30 minutes in a saucepan and about 12 – 15 minutes in a pressure cooker.
4. Drain off the cooked water.
5. Place fava beans, chickpeas, lemon juice, garlic, tahini, salt, thyme and oregano in the food processor bowl or blender and blend until smooth. Add a tablespoon or two of water while blending.
6. Transfer the hummus into a bowl. Garnish with sesame seeds, thyme and garlic.
7. Keep the bowl covered in the refrigerator until ready to serve.

Avocado Hummus

Preparation time: 5 minutes

Cooking time: 0 minutes

Makes: About 1 – 1-½ cups

Ingredients:

- ½ can (from a 15 ounces can) chickpeas, drained or used cooked chickpeas
- 1 ½ tablespoons olive oil + extra to serve
- 1 ½ tablespoons fresh lime juice
- ½ teaspoon ground cumin
- Salt to taste
- Paprika to garnish
- Chopped cilantro or parsley to garnish
- 1 medium (about 6.5 ounces) ripe avocado, peeled, pitted, chopped

Directions:

1. Place chickpeas, oil, lime juice, cumin, salt, and avocado in a blender and blend until smooth.
2. Pour into a bowl. Garnish with cilantro and paprika. Keep the bowl covered in the refrigerator until ready to serve.

Chocolate Hummus

Preparation time: 5 minutes

Cooking time: 0 minutes

Makes: About 1 ¾ cups

Ingredients:

- ¾ cup cooked or canned chickpeas
- 2 tablespoons maple syrup or agave syrup or add more to taste
- ½ teaspoon vanilla extract
- ¼ cup cocoa powder, unsweetened
- 1/8 teaspoon kosher salt
- 2 tablespoons tahini
- A little cooked chickpeas water (or use the water from the can if using canned chickpeas)

To serve: Optional

- Pretzels
- Pineapple wedges
- Strawberries
- Apple slices
- Anything else of your choice

Directions:

1. Place chickpeas, maple syrup, vanilla, tahini, cocoa, and salt in the food processor bowl or blend. Add 1 – 2 tablespoons of the cooked chickpeas water and blend until smooth.
2. Add more water if required, to suit your preference of consistency. Keep the bowl covered in the refrigerator until ready to serve.
3. Serve with any of the suggested serving options.

Edamame Hummus

Preparation time: 5 minutes

Cooking time: 0 minutes

Makes: About 1 ¼ cups

Ingredients:

- 1 cup edamame
- 1 ½ - 2 tablespoons lemon juice
- ½ teaspoon ground cumin
- 2 tablespoons extra-virgin olive oil
- 1 teaspoon chopped garlic
- ¼ teaspoon salt or to taste

Directions:

1. Place edamame, lemon juice, cumin, oil, garlic, and salt in a blender.
2. Blend until smooth. Add a tablespoon or more of water while blending if required.
3. Pour into a bowl. Keep the bowl covered in the refrigerator until ready to serve.

Chapter Four: Falafel Recipes

Classic Falafel

Preparation time: 12 – 24 hours

Cooking time: 20 minutes

Number of servings: 2 – 3

Ingredients:

- ½ pound dried chickpeas, rinsed
- 1 large white onion, chopped
- ¾ teaspoon salt or to taste
- 2 – 3 cloves garlic, minced
- ¼ teaspoon baking soda
- 1/8 cup chopped fresh parsley
- 1 tablespoon flour or chickpea flour
- ½ tablespoon ground cumin
- A pinch ground cardamom
- ½ teaspoon red pepper flakes
- ½ teaspoon ground coriander
- Cayenne pepper to taste
- Black pepper to taste
- ½ teaspoon baking powder (optional)
- Oil to fry, as required

<u>Sesame seeds variation:</u>

- 1 – 2 tablespoons sesame seeds

Turmeric variation:

- ½ teaspoon turmeric powder

Directions:

1. Place chickpeas in a bowl. Pour enough water to cover the chickpeas. Add baking soda and mix well. Cover the bowl and place it in the refrigerator or in a cool and dark area for 12 – 24 hours. If you are soaking it beyond 12 hours, drain the water and pour fresh water to soak.
2. Drain the soaked chickpeas and rinse a couple of times with fresh water.
3. Dry with kitchen towels.
4. Add chickpeas, spices, salt, onion, parsley, and garlic into the food processor bowl. Process until roughly chopped.
5. Give short pulses and process until well incorporated and the chickpeas are very finely chopped. You should not blend it until smooth. The texture should be mostly coarse like sand and a bit pasty.
6. Sprinkle flour and baking powder if using and give short pulses for a few seconds until just incorporated.
7. Transfer into a bowl and cover with a lid. Refrigerate for 4 – 6 hours.

8. Make a falafel from the mixture in the shape of a ball or patty.

9. Place a deep pan over medium-high heat. Pour enough oil to cover the pan by about 3 inches in height.

10. Let the oil heat. When the oil is well heated, but not smoking, about 375° F, place a falafel in the pan. Cook the falafel until golden brown all over. Remove with a slotted spoon and set aside. You will know if the falafel has disintegrated. If it has not disintegrated, great, you are successful in making falafel.

11. In case it disintegrates, no worries. Add a tablespoon or 2 of flour or chickpea flour to the mixture. Try again by frying a small falafel. You should be successful now. If not, you can add some more flour or an egg to hold it together.

12. Now taste the falafel and check it out. If it is very hard or crunchy, it may be that the chickpeas were not processed well, so add the chickpea mixture into the food processor and process until a bit more pasty. Another reason could be that you have not soaked it for long enough so ensure that you soak it for at least 12 hours.

13. Cook the remaining falafels in the similar manner, adding no more than 3 – 4 at a time while frying.

14. Serve with hummus or tahini sauce.

15. To make sesame seeds variation: Once you make the falafel balls or patties, dredge them in sesame seeds before frying.

16. To make turmeric powder variation: Add 1-teaspoon turmeric powder along with the other spices to the food

processor while blending. Carry on with the remaining steps.

Green Falafel

Preparation time: 12 – 24 hours

Cooking time: 20 minutes

Number of servings: 6 – 8

Ingredients:

- 2 cups dried chickpeas, rinsed
- 2 cups chopped fresh cilantro
- 2 cups chopped fresh parsley
- 1 large white onion, chopped (about a cup)
- 1 ¾ teaspoons salt or to taste
- Black pepper to taste
- 1 teaspoon baking soda
- 6 cloves garlic
- 2 small green chili peppers or jalapeño peppers
- 2 teaspoons ground cumin
- 1 teaspoon ground cardamom
- 4 tablespoons chickpea flour
- Oil to fry, as required

Directions:

1. Place chickpeas in a bowl. Pour enough water to cover the chickpeas. . Cover the bowl and place it in the refrigerator or in a cool and dark area for 12 – 24 hours. If you are

soaking it beyond 12 hours, drain the water and pour fresh water to soak.

2. Drain the soaked chickpeas and rinse a couple of times with fresh water.
3. Dry with kitchen towels.
4. Add chickpeas, spices, salt, onion, green chili peppers, cilantro, parsley, and garlic into the food processor bowl. Process until roughly chopped.
5. Give short pulses and process until well incorporated and the chickpeas are very finely chopped. You should not blend it until smooth. The texture should be mostly coarse like sand and a bit pasty.
6. Sprinkle chickpea flour and baking soda and give short pulses for a few seconds until just incorporated. If the mixture is very dry, add a tablespoon or two of water.
7. Transfer into a bowl and cover with a lid. Refrigerate for 4 – 6 hours.
8. Make a falafel from the mixture in the shape of a ball or patty.
9. Place a deep pan over medium-high heat. Pour enough oil to cover the pan by about 3 inches in height.
10. Let the oil heat. When the oil is well heated, but not smoking, about 375° F, place a falafel in the pan. Cook the falafel until golden brown all over. Remove with a slotted spoon and set aside. You will know if the falafel has disintegrated. If it has not disintegrated, great, you are successful in making falafel.

11. In case it disintegrates, no worries. Add a tablespoon or 2 of chickpea flour to the mixture. Try again by frying a small falafel. You should be successful now. If not, you can add some more flour or an egg to hold it together.
12. Now taste the falafel and check it out. If it is very hard or crunchy, it may be that the chickpeas were not processed well, so add the chickpea mixture into the food processor and process until a bit more pasty. Another reason could be that you have not soaked it for long enough so ensure that you soak it for at least 12 hours.
13. Cook the remaining falafels in the similar manner, adding no more than 3 – 4 at a time while frying.
14. Serve with hummus or tahini sauce.

Fava Bean Falafel

Preparation time: 24 hours

Cooking time: 20 minutes

Number of servings: 2 – 3

Ingredients:

- ½ pound dried falafel, rinsed
- 1 large white onion, chopped
- 1 small leek, quartered
- ¾ teaspoon salt or to taste
- 2 – 3 cloves garlic, minced
- ¼ teaspoon baking soda
- 1/8 cup chopped fresh parsley
- 1/8 cup chopped fresh dill
- 1/8 cup chopped fresh cilantro
- 1 tablespoon flour or chickpea flour
- ½ tablespoon ground cumin
- A pinch ground cardamom
- ½ teaspoon red pepper flakes
- ½ teaspoon ground coriander
- 1 teaspoon cayenne pepper to taste
- Black pepper to taste
- ½ teaspoon baking powder (optional)
- 4 teaspoons sesame seeds
- Oil to fry, as required

Directions:

1. Place fava beans in a bowl. Pour enough water to cover the fava beans. Add baking soda and mix well. Cover the bowl and place it in the refrigerator or in a cool and dark area for 24 hours. Do not soak for less time than this.
2. Change the water after 12 hours of soaking.
3. Drain the soaked fava beans and rinse a couple of times with fresh water. Now peel the fava beans.
4. Add fava beans, spice, salt, onion, leek, cilantro, dill, parsley, and garlic into the food processor bowl. Process until roughly chopped.
5. Give short pulses and process until well incorporated and the fava beans are very finely chopped. You should not blend it until smooth. The texture should be mostly coarse like sand and a bit pasty.
6. Sprinkle flour and baking powder if using and give short pulses for a few seconds until just incorporated.
7. Transfer into a bowl. Sprinkle sesame seeds and mix well. Cover with a lid. Refrigerate for 4 – 6 hours.
8. Make a falafel from the mixture in the shape of a ball or patty.
9. Place a deep pan over medium-high heat. Pour enough oil to cover the pan by about 3 inches in height.
10. Let the oil heat. When the oil is well heated, but not smoking, about 375° F, place a falafel in the pan. Cook the falafel until golden brown all over. Remove with a slotted spoon and set aside. You will know if the falafel has

disintegrated. If it has not disintegrated, great, you are successful in making falafel.

11. In case it disintegrates, no worries. Add a tablespoon or 2 of flour or chickpea flour to the mixture. Try again by frying a small falafel. You should be successful now. If not, you can add some more flour or an egg to hold it together.

12. Now taste the falafel and check it out. If it is very hard or crunchy, it may be that the fava beans were not processed well, so add it into the food processor and process until a bit more pasty.

13. Cook the remaining falafels in the similar manner, adding no more than 3 – 4 at a time while frying.

14. Serve with hummus or tahini sauce.

Black Olive Falafel

Preparation time: minutes

Cooking time: minutes

Number of servings:

Ingredients:

- 1 cup dried chickpeas, rinsed
- ½ medium yellow onion, chopped
- ½ cup pitted black kalamata olives
- ½ tablespoon coriander seeds
- ¾ teaspoon kosher salt or to taste
- Black pepper to taste
- 2 cloves garlic
- ¼ teaspoon ground cumin
- 1 – 2 tablespoons chickpea flour
- Oil to fry, as required

Directions:

1. Place chickpeas in a bowl. Pour enough water to cover the chickpeas. Cover the bowl and place it in the refrigerator or in a cool and dark area for 12 – 24 hours. If you are soaking it beyond 12 hours, drain the water and pour fresh water to soak.

2. Drain the soaked chickpeas and rinse a couple of times with fresh water.

3. Dry with kitchen towels.

4. Add chickpeas, spices, salt, onion, olives, and garlic into the food processor bowl. Process until roughly chopped.

5. Give short pulses and process until well incorporated and the chickpeas are very finely chopped. You should not blend it until smooth. The texture should be mostly coarse like sand and a bit pasty.

6. Sprinkle chickpea flour only if the mixture is wet and give short pulses for a few seconds until just incorporated. If the mixture is very dry, add a tablespoon or two of water.

7. Transfer into a bowl and cover with a lid. Refrigerate for 4 – 6 hours.

8. Make a falafel from the mixture in the shape of a ball or patty.

9. Place a deep pan over medium-high heat. Pour enough oil to cover the pan by about 3 inches in height.

10. Let the oil heat. When the oil is well heated, but not smoking, about 375° F, place a falafel in the pan. Cook the falafel until golden brown all over. Remove with a slotted spoon and set aside. You will know if the falafel has disintegrated. If it has not disintegrated, great, you are successful in making falafel.

11. In case it disintegrates, no worries. Add a tablespoon or 2 of chickpea flour to the mixture. Try again by frying a small falafel. You should be successful now. If not, you can add some more flour or an egg to hold it together.

12. Now taste the falafel and check it out. If it is very hard or crunchy, it may be that the chickpeas were not processed well, so add the chickpea mixture into the food processor and process until a bit more pasty. Another reason could be that you have not soaked it for long enough so ensure that you soak it for at least 12 hours.

13. Cook the remaining falafels in the similar manner, adding no more than 3 – 4 at a time while frying.

14. Serve with hummus or tahini sauce

Red Lentil Falafel

Preparation time: 2 – 3 hours

Cooking time: 20 minutes

Number of servings: 6 - 8

Ingredients:

- 2 cups dried red lentils, picked
- 6 cloves garlic, peeled
- 2 green chilies, deseeded, chopped
- 1 ½ teaspoons salt or to taste
- 2 small onions, chopped
- ½ cup fresh cilantro
- 2 teaspoons minced ginger
- 1 teaspoon ground cumin
- 1 tablespoon chickpea flour or flour or more if required
- Paprika to taste (optional)
- Oil to fry, as required

Directions:

1. Rinse the red lentils in water a few times until the water is clear.
2. Pour water into the bowl to cover the lentils. Let it soak for 2 – 3 hours.
3. Dry the lentils with kitchen towels.

4. Add lentils, cumin, salt, onions, green chilies, ginger, paprika, and garlic into the food processor bowl. Process until roughly chopped.
5. Give short pulses and process until well incorporated and the chickpeas are very finely chopped. You should not blend it until smooth. The texture should be mostly coarse like sand and a bit pasty.
6. Sprinkle chickpea flour only if the mixture is wet and give short pulses for a few seconds until just incorporated. If the mixture is very dry, add a tablespoon or two of water.
7. Transfer into a bowl and cover with a lid. Refrigerate for 4 – 6 hours.
8. Make a falafel from the mixture in the shape of a ball or patty.
9. Place a deep pan over medium-high heat. Pour enough oil to cover the pan by about 3 inches in height.
10. Let the oil heat. When the oil is well heated, but not smoking, about 375° F, place a falafel in the pan. Cook the falafel until golden brown all over. Remove with a slotted spoon and set aside. You will know if the falafel has disintegrated. If it has not disintegrated, great, you are successful in making falafel.
11. In case it disintegrates, no worries. Add a tablespoon or 2 of chickpea flour to the mixture. Try again by frying a small falafel. You should be successful now. If not, you can add some more flour, a tablespoon at a time and mix well each time.

12. Cook the remaining falafels in the similar manner, adding no more than 3 – 4 at a time while frying.
13. Serve with hummus or tahini sauce.

Beet and Chickpea Falafel

Preparation time: 12 – 24 hours

Cooking time: 20 minutes

Number of servings: 8 – 10

Ingredients:

- 1 tablespoon olive oil
- 2 teaspoons ground coriander and 2 teaspoons ground cumin
- 2 onions, chopped
- 2 cans (14.5 ounces each) chickpeas, rinsed, drained
- 1 cup breadcrumbs
- 1 tablespoon tahini
- 4 teaspoons cornstarch
- 1 cup breadcrumbs
- 1 teaspoon salt or to taste
- 4 raw beets, peeled, grated

Directions:

1. Pour olive oil into a skillet and heat over medium heat. When oil is hot, add onion and cook until pink.
2. Stir in coriander and cumin and cook for a few seconds until fragrant.

3. Turn off the heat. Add the onion mixture into the food processor.
4. Add chickpeas, beets, and tahini and blend until chickpeas are chopped into smaller pieces.
5. Add breadcrumbs and pulse until coarse in texture. Transfer into a bowl. Add salt and mix well.
6. Transfer into a bowl and cover with a lid. Refrigerate for 4 – 6 hours.
7. Make a falafel from the mixture in the shape of a ball or patty.
8. Place a deep pan over medium-high heat. Pour enough oil to cover the pan by about 3 inches in height.
9. Let the oil heat. When the oil is well heated, but not smoking, about 375° F, place a falafel in the pan. Cook the falafel until golden brown all over. Remove with a slotted spoon and set aside. You will know if the falafel has disintegrated. If it has not disintegrated, great, you are successful in making falafel.
10. If it disintegrates, add some more cornstarch, a teaspoon at a time until the mixture comes together.
11. Serve with hummus or tahini sauce.

Falafel Sandwich

Preparation time: 20 minutes + time to prepare the falafels

Cooking time: 20 minutes to fry falafels

Number of servings: 3

Ingredients:

- 6 – 9 falafels
- Tahini sauce or tzatziki sauce
- 1 tomato, chopped
- ¼ small red onion, sliced
- 3 pita breads
- ¼ cup hummus or more if required
- 1 ½ cups sliced Romaine lettuce or green cabbage
- A handful fresh herbs like cilantro or parsley or dill

Directions:

1. Make falafels using any of the given recipes in this chapter. You may need 3 – 4 falafels per sandwich.
2. Cut off a thin slice from one end of the pitas or you can cut into 2 halves to make 2 pita pockets from each sandwich.
3. Spread hummus inside the pita pockets. Fill the pockets with onion, tomato and lettuce. Spoon some tahini sauce or tzatziki sauce into the pita pockets.
4. Garnish with fresh herbs and serve.

Falafel Salad with Lemon-Tahini Dressing

Preparation time: 10 minutes + to make falafels

Cooking time: 20 minutes to fry falafels

Number of servings: 2

Ingredients:

For salad:

- 8 falafels
- ½ cup packed parsley leaves
- 3 cups sliced Romaine lettuce
- 1 cup quartered grape tomatoes
- 1 cup sliced cucumber or radish

For dressing:

- 1 tablespoon lemon juice
- ½ tablespoon extra-virgin olive oil, divided
- 2 ½ tablespoons tahini
- 2 – 3 tablespoons warm water
- Salt to taste
- Freshly ground pepper to taste

Directions:

1. To make dressing: Whisk together lemon juice, oil, tahini, and water in a bowl. Add salt and pepper to taste.
2. Combine parsley and romaine lettuce in a bowl. Pour half the dressing and stir well.
3. Divide the lettuce into 2 plates.
4. Scatter tomatoes and cucumber over the lettuce. Place 4 falafels on top of each plate. Drizzle remaining dressing on top of the falafels as well as tomatoes and cucumber and serve.

Chapter Five: Salad Recipes

Classic Israeli Salad

Preparation time: 15 minutes

Cooking time: 0 minutes

Number of servings: 2 - 3

Ingredients:

- 1 ½ medium tomatoes, deseeded, cut into ¼ inch squares
- ½ medium red bell pepper, deseeded, cut into ¼ inch squares
- 1 ½ Persian cucumbers or ½ large English cucumber, peel if desired, cut into ¼ inch cubes
- 2 scallions, trimmed, white and light green parts only, thinly sliced
- 1 tablespoon extra-virgin olive oil
- Salt to taste
- 1 tablespoon fresh lemon juice
- Freshly ground pepper to taste

Directions:

1. Add tomatoes, bell pepper, cucumber, and scallions into a bowl and toss well.
2. Add oil, salt, pepper, and lemon juice and toss well.
3. Serve immediately.

Israeli Bell Pepper Salad

Preparation time: 20 minutes

Cooking time: 0 minutes

Number of servings: 4

Ingredients:

- 1/3 cup chopped flat-leaf parsley
- 1 medium yellow bell pepper, diced (½ inch dice)
- 1 medium red bell pepper, diced (½ inch dice)
- 1 medium green bell pepper, diced (½ inch dice)
- 1 medium onion, thinly sliced
- ½ cup chopped mint leaves

For dressing:

- 4 tablespoons extra-virgin olive oil
- Kosher salt to taste
- 2 teaspoons za'atar spice blend
- 4 tablespoons fresh lemon juice

Directions:

1. To make dressing: Add oil, salt, za'atar spice, and lemon juice into a bowl and whisk well.
2. Add bell peppers, onion, parsley, and mint and toss well.
3. Set aside the salad for a while for the flavors to blend.

Israeli Salad with Za'atar Dressing

Preparation time: 20 minutes

Cooking time: 0 minutes

Number of servings: 4

Ingredients:

- ½ cup diced Persian cucumber English cucumber, peel if desired, cut into ¼ inch cubes
- ¼ cup red onion, diced
- ¾ cup red bell pepper, deseeded, cut into ¼ inch squares
- ½ cup halved cherry tomatoes
- ½ cup diced radish, cut into ¼ inch cubes
- ½ cup cubed feta cheese
- ¼ cup finely chopped parsley

For dressing:

- 2 tablespoons extra-virgin olive oil
- Salt to taste
- ½ teaspoon za'atar spice blend
- 1 ½ tablespoons fresh lemon juice
- Freshly cracked pepper to taste

Directions:

1. Add tomatoes, bell pepper, cucumber, radish, parsley, and onion into a bowl and toss well.
2. To make dressing: Add oil, salt, pepper, za'atar spice, and lemon juice into a bowl and whisk well.
3. Set aside the dressing for a while for the flavors to blend.
4. Toss well. Add feta cheese and toss lightly.
5. Serve immediately.

Classic Jewish Deli Chicken Salad

Preparation time: 10 minutes

Cooking time: 0 minutes

Number of servings: 4 – 5

Ingredients:

- ½ cut-up whole chicken, cooked, shredded
- 2 carrots, peeled, grated
- 2 stalks celery, finely diced
- ½ tablespoon grated onion or more to suit your taste
- ¼ - ½ cup Hellmann's mayonnaise
- Salt to taste
- ½ can jellied cranberry sauce (optional)
- Pepper to taste

Directions:

1. Place chicken, carrot, and celery in a bowl and toss well.
2. Add onion, mayonnaise, salt, pepper, and cranberry sauce if using and mix well. Keep the bowl covered in the refrigerator until use.
3. Serve.

Israeli Couscous Salad with Vegetables

Preparation time: 10 minutes

Cooking time: 10 minutes

Number of servings: 2

Ingredients:

- 1 cup Israeli couscous
- ½ veggie bouillon cube
- 1 cup water
- 5 Greek kalamata olives, diced
- ½ tablespoon olive oil
- 1/8 red onions, diced
- ¼ cucumber, diced
- Salt and pepper to taste

Directions:

1. To make broth: Dissolve bouillon cube in water.
2. Place a pot over medium heat. Add oil and allow it to heat. When the oil is hot, add couscous and cook until light brown, stirring constantly.
3. Add broth and stir. When it starts boiling, lower the heat and cook until dry.
4. Turn off the heat and fluff with a fork. Transfer into a bowl. Let it cool.

5. Add olives, onion, and cucumber and toss well.
6. Divide into bowls and serve.

Israeli Couscous Salad with Chicken

Preparation time: 15 minutes

Cooking time: 20 minutes

Number of servings: 2

Ingredients:

- 1 chicken breast, boneless, skinless
- 1 ½ tablespoons extra-virgin olive oil
- ½ tablespoon olive oil
- 1/8 teaspoon red pepper flakes
- Salt to taste
- Pepper to taste
- 1 cup water
- ½ cup Israeli couscous
- ¼ cup halved yellow grape tomatoes
- 1/8 cup thinly sliced red onions
- ¼ cup sliced Greek kalamata olives
- Juice of ½ lemon
- 1 clove garlic, peeled, crushed
- ¼ English cucumber, peeled, diced
- 1 ounce feta, cubed
- ½ tablespoon red wine vinegar
- 1/8 cup chopped parsley or basil leaves

Directions:

1. Whisk together half the extra-virgin olive oil, lemon juice, red pepper flakes, garlic, and thyme leaves in a bowl.
2. Add chicken and turn it over to coat well. Cover and set it aside for a while for the flavors to meld.
3. Place a pot over medium heat. Add olive oil. When the oil is hot, add couscous and stir frequently until light brown.
4. Add water and stir. When it comes to a boil, lower the heat and cover with a lid. Cook until dry.
5. When done, fluff with a fork. Transfer into a bowl. Let it cool.
6. Meanwhile cook the chicken:
7. Add cucumber, tomato, feta, onion, parsley, and olives into a bowl and toss well.
8. Add couscous and toss well.
9. Whisk together remaining extra-virgin olive oil, salt, and pepper in a bowl. Pour over the salad. Toss well and keep it aside.
10. Cook the chicken on a grill or in a grill pan. Take out the chicken from the marinade and sprinkle salt and pepper over it. Cook over the grill or in a pan over medium-high heat for 5 minutes on each side and cook through inside.
11. Let the chicken rest for 5 minutes. Cut into slices diagonally.
12. Divide the salad into bowls. Top with chicken slices and serve.

Israeli Chickpea Salad

Preparation time: 10 minutes

Cooking time: 0 minutes

Number of servings: 2 – 3

Ingredients:

- ½ can (from a 14.5 ounces can) chickpeas, drained
- ½ cucumber, peeled, deseeded, diced
- 1 ½ large ripe plum tomatoes, deseeded, diced
- ½ green bell pepper, diced
- 1/8 cup chopped Bermuda onion

For dressing:

- 1 ½ tablespoons lemon juice
- Salt to taste
- 2 tablespoons olive oil
- ¼ teaspoon pepper or to taste
- 2 teaspoons white vinegar

Directions:

1. Whisk together lemon juice, salt, oil, pepper and vinegar in a bowl to make the dressing.

2. Add chickpeas and vegetables and toss well.

3. Serve.

Tabbouleh

Preparation time: 30 minutes

Cooking time: 0 minutes

Number of servings: 2 – 3

Ingredients:

- 2 – 3 scallions, chopped
- 1 teaspoon ground cumin
- 1/8 cup fresh lemon juice or to taste
- 2 – 3 tablespoons olive oil
- 1/8 cup chopped fresh mint
- ½ bunch fresh, flat-leaf parsley, chopped
- 1 cup chopped grape tomatoes
- Kosher salt to taste
- 6 – 8 tablespoons fine bulgur

Directions:

1. Soak bulgur in a bowl of hot water for 15 minutes. Place a strainer over a bowl. Pour the bulgur into the strainer.

2. Let the drained bulgur remain in the strainer for about 30 minutes. Transfer bulgur into a bowl.
3. Add lemon juice, olive oil, salt, and cumin and stir until well combined. Cover and set aside for about 45 minutes, for the flavors to mix up.
4. Add mint, parsley, scallions, and tomatoes and toss well.
5. Garnish with some mint or parsley if desired and serve.

Israeli Fruit Salad

Preparation time: 10 minutes

Cooking time: 10 minutes

Number of servings: 4 - 5

Ingredients:

- 1 ripe plum, pitted, sliced (do not peel)
- ¼ cup pitted, finely chopped dates
- ¼ cup pomegranate arils + extra to garnish
- 1/8 cup finely chopped mint leaves + extra to garnish
- 1 red or green ripe pear, cored, cubed (do not peel)
- ¼ cup thinly sliced fresh figs
- Zest of ½ lime, grated
- Juice of ½ lime, grated
- ½ tablespoon honey

Directions:

1. Combine all the fresh fruits in a bowl. Add dates, mint, lime juice, lime zest, and honey and mix well.
2. Garnish with mint and serve.

Eggplant and Red Pepper Salad

Preparation time: 35 minutes

Cooking time: 60 minutes

Number of servings: 6

Ingredients:

- 1 large eggplant, trimmed, cut into ½ inch thick slices
- 1 red or yellow bell pepper, cored, cut into 1 inch squares
- ½ can (from a 15 ounces can) tomato sauce
- ½ teaspoon ground cumin
- ½ teaspoon sugar
- ¼ teaspoon black pepper
- 3 tablespoons olive oil
- 2 cloves garlic, peeled, smashed, finely chopped
- ½ cup water
- Sea salt to taste
- ¼ teaspoon crushed red pepper flakes
- 1 tablespoon chopped parsley (optional)

Directions:

1. Take a peeler and peel the eggplant lengthwise once. Next to it leave the skin on. Repeat this alternate peeling and not peeling. In other words the eggplant is peeled in one part and next part it is unpeeled. It should be this way all

throughout the eggplant. Now chop the eggplant into 1-inch chunks.

2. Pour a tablespoon of oil into a skillet and place the skillet over medium heat. Add bell pepper and cook for a couple of minutes and garlic and mix well.
3. Cook for about a minute or until fragrant. Transfer into a bowl.
4. Add remaining oil into the skillet. When oil is hot, add eggplant and cook until brown all over.
5. Whisk together tomato sauce, salt, sugar, cumin, water, crushed red pepper, and pepper in a bowl.
6. Pour the sauce mixture into the skillet. Add the bell pepper into the skillet. Cover the skillet, leaving a small part open for the steam to escape and simmer on low heat for about 30 – 40 minutes until thick. Stir occasionally.
7. Turn off the heat. This salad can be served hot or cold. This tastes great with bread that is freshly baked.
8. Garnish with parsley and serve.

Roasted Cauliflower Salad with Lemon Tahini Dressing

Preparation time: 15 minutes

Cooking time: 35 minutes

Number of servings: 8

Ingredients:

- 2 heads cauliflower, cut into bite size florets
- 4 tablespoons olive oil
- 1 bunch parsley, chopped
- 1 red onion, cut into ¼ inch thick slices
- Salt to taste
- Pepper to taste

For dressing:

- 2/3 cup tahini
- ½ cup lemon juice
- 1 teaspoon ground cumin
- ½ teaspoon salt
- 2/3 cup water
- 4 cloves garlic, peeled, minced
- ½ teaspoon cayenne pepper

For spicy chickpeas:

- 2 cans (15 ounces each) chickpeas, drained, rinsed
- 1 teaspoon smoked paprika
- ¼ teaspoon cayenne pepper
- Pepper to taste
- 2 tablespoons olive oil
- ½ teaspoon garlic powder
- 3 cups chopped parsley
- Salt to taste

Directions:

1. Set the temperature of the oven to 400° F and preheat the oven.
2. Place cauliflower and onions on a baking sheet. Pour oil over them. Add salt and pepper to taste and mix well.
3. Spread it evenly all over the baking sheet and place it in the oven. Set the timer for about 40 – 45 minutes, until cooked inside and brown on the outside. Stir the vegetables every 15 minutes. Make sure to spread it all over the baking sheet each time.
4. Once ready, take out the baking sheet and let it cool for a few minutes.
5. While the vegetables are roasting, cook the chickpeas and make the dressing:
6. Blend together tahini, garlic, lemon juice, water, salt, cayenne, and cumin in a blender until very smooth. Pour the dressing into a bowl and chill until use.

7. Dry the chickpeas by patting with paper towels. Place a skillet over medium heat.
8. Add oil and swirl the pan to spread oil. Add chickpeas, salt and spices and cook until dry and a bit crisp. Turn off the heat. Let it cool for a few minutes.
9. To make salad: Place roasted vegetables in a bowl. Add chickpeas and parsley and toss well.
10. Pour dressing over the salad. Mix well and serve. This salad can be served warm or at room temperature or cold.

Beet Chickpea and Walnut Salad

Preparation time: 10 minutes + soaking time

Cooking time: 20 minutes + marinating time

Number of servings: 7 – 8

Ingredients:

- 6 medium beets, trimmed
- 4 shallots, thinly sliced
- 2 cups cooked or canned chickpeas
- 4 – 6 cups chopped lettuce
- A handful chopped walnuts

For dressing:

- 1 cup fresh orange juice
- 4 cloves garlic, peeled
- ½ cup lemon juice
- 8 walnut halves
- 4 teaspoons sugar

Directions:

1. Boil the beets in a pot of water until tender. Drain and allow it to cool completely.
2. Peel and cut the beets into bite size pieces.

3. Place beets, chickpeas, and shallots in a bowl and toss well.
4. For dressing: Soak the walnuts for a couple of hours in water. Blend together the dressing ingredients in a blender until smooth. Pour into the bowl of salad. Mix well.
5. Cover the bowl and let it marinate for 4 – 24 hours.
6. Add lettuce just before serving. Toss well. Sprinkle walnuts on top and serve.

Parsley Salad with Pine Nuts and Lemon-Tahini Dressing

Preparation time: 10 minutes; Cooking time: 3 – 4 minutes

Number of servings: 2

Ingredients:

- 1/8 cup pine nuts
- 3 teaspoons fresh lemon juice
- 1 tablespoon water
- 2 cups flat-leaf parsley leaves
- 2 tablespoons tahini paste, at room temperature
- ½ small clove garlic, minced
- Salt to taste
- 2 scallions, cut into thin slices crosswise
- Freshly ground pepper to taste

Directions:

1. Combine tahini, water, lemon juice, garlic, pepper, and salt in a bowl. Add more water if the dressing is too thick.
2. Add pine nuts into a skillet and place the skillet over medium heat. Shake the pan occasionally and toast the nuts until they turn golden brown.
3. Turn off the heat and place them on a plate to cool completely.

4. Place scallions, pine nuts, and parsley in a bowl and toss
    well. Add dressing and fold gently.

Chapter Six: Miscellaneous Israeli Recipes

Israeli Spice Chicken

Preparation time: 20 minutes

Cooking time: 15 minutes

Number of servings: 2

Ingredients:

For spice rub:

- ¾ tablespoon sweet paprika
- ½ teaspoon dried oregano
- ½ teaspoon crushed red pepper flakes
- ¾ tablespoon ground cumin
- ½ teaspoon ground coriander
- ¾ teaspoon coarse kosher salt

For chicken:

- Extra-virgin olive oil to drizzle
- 2 boneless, skinless chicken breasts
- Warm pita bread or flatbread

For dressing:

- 1 ½ tablespoons extra-virgin olive oil
- ¼ teaspoon ground cumin

- ¼ teaspoon crushed red pepper flakes
- Juice of ½ lemon
- ¼ teaspoon ground coriander
- Kosher salt to taste

<u>For tomato relish:</u>

- 1 orange or yellow tomato, deseeded, chopped
- 1 ½ vine rip or small red tomatoes, deseeded, chopped
- ¼ cup chopped flat-leaf parsley
- ½ small sweet onion, thinly sliced

Directions:

1. To make spice rub: Combine all the spices and salt in a bowl. You can use all of it or use as much as you think is needed. If you are not using all of it, store the remaining rub in an airtight container in a cool place. It can last for 6 months.
2. Drizzle chicken all over the chicken and place it in a container.
3. Sprinkle the spice rub over the chicken and rub it into it. Let it rest for 10 minutes.
4. Preheat your grill to medium heat. Place chicken on the grill and grill for 6 – 7 minutes. Turn the chicken over and cook the other side for 6 – 7 minutes.
5. Combine tomatoes, parsley, and onion in a bowl.
6. Whisk together all the dressing ingredients in a bowl and drizzle over the salad. Toss well. Let it rest for 10 minutes.

7. Cut off a thin slice from one end of the pita bread to make pockets.

8. Fill the pockets with pita bread and tomato relish and serve.

Herbed Tahini Grilled Lamb Chops with Israeli Couscous

Preparation time: 30 minutes

Cooking time: 30 minutes

Number of servings: 2 – 3

Ingredients:

<u>For herbed tahini sauce:</u>

- ¼ cup tahini
- ¼ cup fresh flat-leaf parsley leaves
- ¼ cup fresh cilantro leaves and tender stems
- Juice of ½ lemon
- Zest of ½ lemon, grated
- ¼ teaspoon ground cumin
- Salt to taste
- ½ tablespoon olive oil
- 1 clove garlic, peeled,
- Cayenne pepper to taste (optional)
- ¼ cup water

<u>For couscous:</u>

- 1 teaspoon olive oil
- ¼ teaspoon black pepper
- ¼ teaspoon onion powder
- ¼ teaspoon garlic powder
- ¾ cup Israeli couscous
- ¾ cup + 1/8 cup chicken or vegetable broth
- Salt to taste
- ½ tablespoon butter

<u>For lamb chops:</u>

- 1 pound lamb chops (1 inch thick)
- Salt to taste
- ½ tablespoon olive oil
- Black pepper to taste

Directions:

1. To make herbed tahini sauce: Place the sauce ingredients in a blender and blend until smooth. Taste the sauce and adjust the salt if required. The sauce should be of pouring consistency so add more water if required while blending.
2. To make couscous: Place a pot over medium heat. Add oil and allow it to heat. When the oil is hot, add couscous and cook until light brown, stirring constantly.
3. Add spices and salt and mix well.

4. Add broth and stir. When it starts boiling, lower the heat and cook until dry.
5. Remove from heat. Add butter and fluff with a fork.
6. To make lamb chops: Brush oil over the lamb chops. Sprinkle salt and pepper to taste.
7. Preheat your grill to medium-high heat. Place lamb chops on the grill and grill for 2 – 3 minutes. Turn the lamb chops over and cook the other side for 2 – 3 minutes.
8. Take out the lamb chops from the grill and place on a plate. Let it sit for 5 minutes.
9. Serve lamb chops with couscous. Drizzle the herbed tahini sauce on top and serve.

Grilled Steak

Preparation time: 10 minutes

Cooking time: 10 minutes

Number of servings: 2

Ingredients:

- 1 ¼ pounds steak, trimmed
- ½ tablespoon ground turmeric
- ½ tablespoon ground black pepper
- A pinch cayenne pepper
- ½ tablespoon ground cumin
- ½ tablespoon ground coriander
- ½ tablespoon kosher salt

Serving options:

- Rice
- Cooked potatoes or corn
- Any side dish of your choice

Directions:

1. Prick holes all over the steak using a fork.
2. Combine all the spices and salt in a bowl. Rub this mixture all over the steak.

3. Preheat your grill to medium-high heat. Spray the steak on both sides with some cooking spray.
4. Place steak on the grill and grill for 3 – 5 minutes. Turn the steak over and cook the other side for 3 – 5 minutes.
5. Take out the steak from the grill and place on your cutting board. Let it sit for 5 minutes. Cut the steak into thin slices.
6. Serve steak with any of the suggested serving options.

Israeli Kofta Kabobs

Preparation time: 25 minutes

Cooking time: 30 minutes

Number of servings: 6

Ingredients:

- 1 pound ground beef
- ½ pound ground lamb
- 1 cup Italian breadcrumbs
- ½ large bunch cilantro, minced
- 2 large onions, minced
- 2 eggs
- ½ teaspoon curry powder
- 1/8 teaspoon hot paprika
- ½ teaspoon paprika
- ½ tablespoon chicken bouillon powder
- ½ teaspoon pepper
- 1 ½ teaspoons sea salt

Directions:

1. Set the temperature of the oven to 350° F and preheat the oven.
2. Combine breadcrumbs, cilantro, spices, onion, eggs, and salt in a bowl.

3. Add meat and mix well. As you mix, massage the contents well. If the mixture is very sticky or runny, add some more breadcrumbs.
4. Take about 3 tablespoons of the mixture and wrap it around a skewer. Place on a baking sheet. This is a kabob. Make the remaining kabobs similarly with the remaining meat mixture.
5. Place the baking sheet in the oven and set the timer for 30 minutes or until cooked. Turn the kabobs over after about 15 minutes of baking.
6. Serve hot kabobs with some salad and hot cooked rice if desired.

Jerusalem Mixed Grill

Preparation time: 15 minutes

Cooking time: 20 minutes

Number of servings: 2

Ingredients:

- 7 ounces boneless chicken breast, chopped
- 1.8 ounce chicken heart, chopped
- 7 ounces chicken liver, chopped
- ½ large onion, sliced
- 2 tablespoons extra-virgin olive oil
- ½ tablespoon grated garlic
- ½ teaspoon curry powder
- ½ teaspoon turmeric powder
- ½ teaspoon ground cumin
- ½ teaspoon coriander powder
- ¾ teaspoon paprika powder

Directions:

1. Pour oil into a skillet and heat it over medium heat. Add onion and sauté for a couple of minutes.
2. Mix together all the spices in a bowl. Add half this mixture into the skillet and mix it up well with the onion.
3. Transfer the onion onto a plate.

4. Add garlic into the skillet and stir-fry for about a minute, until you get a nice aroma.
5. Stir in chicken breast, heart, chicken liver, and remaining spices in the skillet.
6. Cook covered until the liquid in the skillet dries up.
7. Add onion and mix well. Turn off the heat and serve immediately with pita bread and hummus.

Israeli Turmeric Rice

Preparation time: 5 minutes

Cooking time: 20 minutes

Number of servings: 2

Ingredients:

- 1 cup long grain rice
- 1 teaspoon ground ginger
- 1 teaspoon turmeric powder
- ½ teaspoon salt or to taste
- 2 tablespoons oil
- 2 ¼ cups vegetable stock
- ½ teaspoon pepper

For fried mint leaves

- ½ bunch mint leaves
- ½ tablespoon olive oil

Directions:

1. Place a pot over medium heat. Add oil and swirl the pot so that the oil spreads.
2. Let the oil heat. Add rice and stir-fry for a few minutes until rice turns opaque.

3. Add pepper, ground ginger, and turmeric and mix well. Stir for about 10 – 15 seconds.
4. Add the rest of the ingredients and stir. When it begins to boil, lower the heat and simmer until rice is cooked.
5. Turn off the heat. Fluff the rice with a fork.
6. To make fried mint leaves: Pour oil into a small pan and let it heat over medium heat.
7. Once oil is hot, add mint leaves and stir. Cook until the leaves turn crisp, turn occasionally.
8. Serve hot rice garnished with fried mint leaves.

Israeli Lentil Soup

Preparation time: 15 minutes

Cooking time: 30 – 40 minutes

Number of servings: 8 – 10

Ingredients:

- 2 cups dried lentils, rinsed well, soaked in water for a while
- 4 carrots, shredded
- 4 bay leaves
- 2 cups chopped onions
- ¼ cup chopped fresh parsley
- 4 cloves garlic, peeled, minced
- 8 celery ribs, shredded
- Salt to taste or garlic salt to taste
- 1 teaspoon ground cumin
- Pepper to taste
- 4 tablespoons lemon juice
- 6 cups chicken broth
- ½ teaspoon dried thyme
- 2 cups cooked, diced chicken or turkey
- 6 cups water
- ½ teaspoon turmeric powder or curry powder (optional)

Directions:

1. Place lentils, bay leaves, vegetables, spices, salt, water, and broth in a large soup pot.
2. Place the soup pot over high heat.
3. When it starts boiling, lower the heat and cover with a lid. Cook until lentils are soft.
4. Add lemon juice and chicken and mix well. Heat thoroughly.
5. Ladle into soup bowls and serve.

Za'atar Crusted Gefilte Fish

Preparation time: 5 minutes

Cooking time: 1 hour and 10 minutes

Number of servings: 3 – 4

Ingredients:

- 2 loaves frozen gefilte fish
- 1 teaspoon salt
- 2/3 cup olive oil
- Water as required
- ½ cup za'atar spice blend
- 1/8 teaspoon pepper
- 2 teaspoons wasabi powder
- ½ cup mayonnaise

Directions:

1. Set the temperature of the oven to 350° F and preheat the oven.
2. Add salt, pepper, za'atar spice blend and oil in a bowl and stir. Spread this mixture all over the frozen fish and place them in a baking dish.
3. Place the baking dish in the oven and set the temperature for 1 hour.

4. Raise the temperature of the oven to 425° F and bake for another 10 minutes or until brown on top.
5. To make wasabi aioli: Make a paste of wasabi powder following the instructions on the package.
6. Add mayonnaise and mix well.
7. Serve fish warm or at room temperature with wasabi aioli.

Chicken and Veggie Stuffed Pita

Preparation time: 25 minutes

Cooking time: 12 minutes

Number of servings: 2

Ingredients:

- 2 boneless chicken thighs
- ¾ tablespoon olive oil or more if required
- 1 Portobello mushrooms, sliced
- Salt to taste
- Pepper to taste
- ½ small bunch asparagus, chopped
- 1 teaspoon za'atar spice blend or to taste
- Israeli hot sauce schug to taste
- Tahini sauce to serve
- ¼ cup chopped parsley
- 2 pita breads to serve, halved

Directions:

1. Pour oil into a pan and place the pan over medium heat and let the oil heat.
2. Season chicken with salt and pepper and place in the pan. Cook until the underside is golden brown, about 4

minutes. Turn the chicken over and cook the other side until golden brown.

3. Stir in mushrooms and asparagus. Increase the heat to high heat and cook until the vegetables are tender.

4. Turn off the heat. Sprinkle a generous amount of za'atar over the chicken and vegetables and stuff it inside the pita pockets. Spoon some schug, tahini sauce and parsley into the pita pockets and serve.

Matzoballs Chicken Soup

Preparation time: 20 minutes

Cooking time: 40 minutes

Number of servings: 4

Ingredients:

For soup:

- 1 – 1 ½ pounds cut up chicken, skin-on
- 1 large onion, halved, sliced
- ½ bunch parsley, chopped
- ½ bunch dill, chopped
- 2 parsley roots, peeled, halved if large
- 3 medium carrots, halved, sliced
- Kosher salt to taste
- ½ tablespoon black peppercorns

For Matzoballs:

- ½ cup matzomeal
- ½ teaspoon baking powder
- A large pinch pepper
- ½ teaspoon minced fresh dill
- 2 eggs
- 1/8 teaspoon salt
- 1 ½ tablespoons vegetable oil or schmaltz

Directions:

1. Place chicken in a soup pot and pour enough cold water to cover the chicken. Place the saucepan over medium heat.
2. Soon, as the water starts boiling, scum will start floating on the surface of the water. Do not remove it and let it cook for about 20 minutes. Turn off the heat.
3. Drain the broth into a bowl. Rinse the chicken well and clean the pot of any scum.
4. Place carrots, onion, herbs, chicken, pepper, and salt into the pot. Pour enough cold water to cover the ingredients in the pot. Place the pot over high heat.
5. When water starts boiling, lower the heat to medium-low heat and simmer for about 1-½ hours.
6. To make Matzoballs: Combine matzomeal, baking powder, salt, pepper, dill, eggs, and oil in a bowl.
7. Make small balls of the mixture and keep them on a plate. Slide them into the simmering soup, one at a time. Cook for 25 minutes if you want heavy Matzoballs and for about 35 minutes if you want light Matzoballs.
8. Serve soup in bowls, making sure to serve meatballs, chicken, and vegetables in each bowl.

Israeli Eggplant

Preparation time: 30 minutes

Cooking time: 30 minutes

Number of servings: 2

Ingredients:

Ingredients:

- 1 medium eggplant, trimmed, cut into ½ inch thick half-moon slices
- ½ cup chopped onion
- 4 tablespoons chopped parsley
- 1 tablespoon kosher salt
- ½ cup chopped red bell pepper
- ½ teaspoon paprika
- ½ tablespoon ground coriander
- 2 tablespoons sherry vinegar
- ½ tablespoon lemon juice
- 3 – 4 tablespoons olive oil or more if required

Directions:

1. Sprinkle salt over the eggplant slices and place in a colander. Place the colander over a bowl. You can also

place them over layers of paper towels. Let the moisture drain for 30 minutes.

2. Rinse the eggplant slices under running water. Drain well. Dry the slices with paper towels.
3. Place a pan over medium-high heat. Pour about 3 – 4 tablespoons of oil into the pan.
4. When the oil is well heated and not smoking, about 375° F, place eggplant slices.
5. Cook until golden brown, turning occasionally. Remove with a slotted spoon and place on a plate lined with paper towels.
6. Add a little more oil in the pan and take out the rest. Add red pepper and onion into the pan and stir-fry for 3 – 5 minutes, until tender. Add spices and mix well. Cook for about a minute or two until you get a nice aroma.
7. Add eggplant and vinegar and mix well. Cook until dry. Turn off the heat.
8. Add lemon juice and stir.
9. Garnish with parsley and serve it cold or warm.

Israeli Lamb Stew with Dill and Olives

Preparation time: 15 minutes

Cooking time: 30 - 40 minutes

Number of servings: 3

Ingredients:

- ¼ cup extra-virgin olive oil
- 1 onion, finely chopped
- Salt to taste
- ½ cup beef stock
- ¾ pound spinach, chopped
- 4 green onions, white part only, finely chopped
- 1 ½ pounds lamb shoulder or stew meat, cut into 2 inch cubes
- ½ teaspoon turmeric powder
- 1 cup peeled, diced, potatoes
- Freshly ground pepper to taste
- 6 tablespoons lemon juice
- 1 bunch celery, use only leaves, finely chopped
- 1 tablespoon minced fresh dill
- ½ cup pitted, halved, green olives

Directions:

1. Pour tablespoon of oil into a heatproof casserole and place over medium heat. When the oil is hot, add onion and lamb meat and cook until brown all over, stirring occasionally.
2. Stir in salt, pepper and turmeric. Stir for about 8 – 10 seconds.
3. Pour beef stock and lemon juice. Mix well.
4. Lower the heat and cook covered, for 10 – 12 minutes. Stir often.
5. Add 3 tablespoons of oil into a heavy bottomed skillet. Place the skillet over medium heat. Add celery, spinach, and green onions Cook until the greens wilt.
6. Transfer into the casserole dish and mix well.
7. Add potatoes, olives, and dill and mix well. Cover and cook until meat and vegetables are tender, about 30 minutes. Stir frequently.
8. Serve over rice or couscous.

St. Peter's Fish with Parsley Sauce

Preparation time: 10 minutes

Cooking time: 15 minutes

Number of servings: 2

Ingredients:

- ½ cup chopped fresh parsley
- 1 tablespoon water + extra to dilute
- Juice of ½ lemon
- 2 St. Peter's fish or bass or trout fillets
- ¼ cup olive oil
- 2 small cloves garlic, chopped
- Salt to taste
- Pepper to taste
- 1 ½ tablespoons flour
- 1/8 cup chopped onion

Directions:

1. Blend together parsley, water, and garlic in a blender until smooth.
2. Transfer into a bowl. Add lemon juice, pepper, and salt and stir. Add a tablespoon or two of water to dilute and stir. Cover and keep it aside.

3. Combine flour, pepper, and salt on a plate. Dredge the fillets in a flour mixture. Shake off extra flour and place on a plate.
4. Pour oil into a heavy bottom skillet and let it heat over medium heat. When oil is hot, place fish in the pan and cook until brown on either side.
5. Remove fish from the pan and place on a preheated serving plate. Keep warm until the sauce is cooked.
6. Remove half the oil from the pan and onions into the pan. Cook until golden brown.
7. Stir in flour. Keep stirring until flour turns light brown. Pour the blended parsley mixture into the pan and stir constantly until thick. When the mixture starts boiling, turn off the heat.
8. Spoon the sauce over the fish and serve.

Israeli Meatballs in Tehina

Preparation time: 15 minutes

Cooking time: 30 – 40 minutes

Number of servings: 4

Ingredients:

- 1 container (8 ounces) Sabra Tehina
- 2 – 3 tablespoons water
- ½ small onion, minced
- ¼ cup breadcrumbs
- A handful chopped parsley + extra to garnish
- ½ teaspoon ground cumin
- 1/8 teaspoon ground ginger and salt to taste
- Freshly ground pepper to taste
- 1 tablespoon canola oil
- 1 pound lean chopped meat
- 2 cloves garlic, minced
- 1 egg, beaten
- ¼ teaspoon ground cinnamon
- ½ teaspoon turmeric powder
- ½ teaspoon paprika + extra to garnish
- 1 tablespoon halved pistachios or pine nuts, toasted

Directions:

1. Combine water and tehina. Keep it aside.
2. Place meat in a bowl. Add onion, breadcrumbs, pepper, salt, turmeric, garlic ginger, egg, cinnamon, and cumin and mix well. Do not over mix.
3. Make small meatballs of the mixture.
4. Place an ovenproof skillet over medium heat. Add oil and swirl the pan to spread oil.
5. Add meatballs into the pan and cook until brown all over. Cook them in batches if required to avoid overcrowding.
6. Transfer the meatballs onto a plate. Clean the pan and add half the tehina into the skillet. Place meatballs in the skillet, over the tehina. Drizzle remaining tehina over the meatballs.
7. Shift the pan into the oven and bake for about 30 minutes or until the meat is cooked through.

Freekeh Vegetable Soup

Preparation time: 15 minutes

Cooking time: 45 -60 minutes

Number of servings: 8

Ingredients:

- 2 cups cracked freekeh
- ½ medium kohlrabi, peeled, diced
- 2 cloves garlic, minced
- ½ large onion, diced
- 1 medium carrot, peeled, diced
- 1 medium zucchini, diced
- ½ teaspoon kosher salt to taste
- 4 cups vegetable or chicken broth + extra if required
- 1 teaspoon chopped fresh za'atar or oregano
- Chopped fresh za'atar or chives or parsley to garnish
- Freshly ground pepper to taste
- ½ tablespoon nutritional yeast or ½ parmesan rind (optional)
- Cayenne pepper to taste

Directions:

1. Soak freekeh in a bowl of cold water. Keep it aside for 15 minutes. Drain and rinse well in cold water. Drain finally after rinsing.
2. Pour oil into a soup pot and let it heat over medium heat.
3. When oil is hot, add onion and cook until it turns pink. Stir in kohlrabi and carrots and cook until slightly tender.
4. Add salt and pepper to taste. Stir in the garlic. Keep stirring for about a minute.
5. Add freekeh and mix well. Stir in zucchini, broth, za'atar, cayenne pepper, salt, and Parmesan rind or nutritional yeast.
6. When the soup starts boiling, lower the heat and cook until thick. Do not cover the pot.
7. Discard the Parmesan rind. Add salt and pepper to taste,
8. Ladle into soup bowls. Sprinkle fresh herbs on top. Trickle oil on top and serve.

Lemon Infused Couscous Pearls

Preparation time: 10 minutes

Cooking time: 15 – 20 minutes

Number of servings: 2

Ingredients:

- ½ cup Israeli couscous
- ½ small shallot, finely diced
- ½ cup + 1/8 cup chicken stock or water
- Finely chopped parsley to garnish
- ½ tablespoon butter
- ½ teaspoon grated lemon zest + extra to garnish
- 1/8 cup shredded parmesan cheese + extra to garnish

Directions:

1. Add butter into a small pan. Add shallot and lemon zest and place the pan over medium heat. Let it cook for about 3 minutes, making sure not to brown the ingredients.
2. Add couscous and mix well. Toast for a couple of minutes. Add chicken stock or water and mix well.
3. Add salt and pepper to taste. Cook until dry. Turn off the heat. Take a fork and fluff the couscous.
4. Add Parmesan cheese and stir.

5. Serve in bowls, garnished with lemon zest, parsley, and Parmesan.

Baba Ganoush

Preparation time: 10 minutes

Cooking time: 35 minutes

Number of servings:

Ingredients:

- 2 medium eggplants (2 – 2 ½ pounds in all)
- 4 teaspoons lemon juice or to taste
- 2 tablespoons chopped fresh parsley
- 4 cloves garlic, minced
- 2/3 cup tahini
- Salt to taste
- Olive oil to drizzle

Directions:

1. Set the temperature of the oven to 350° F and preheat the oven.
2. Pierce eggplants all over with a fork.
3. Take a rimmed baking sheet and place the eggplants on it.
4. Place the baking sheet in the oven and roast the eggplants for about 35 minutes or until tender inside. Turn the eggplants every 10 – 12 minutes.

5. When the eggplants are roasted well, remove from the oven and let it cool. Discard the skin.

6. Place the eggplant, garlic, lemon juice, tahini and salt in a food processor. Blend until slightly chunky or the texture you desire.

7. Transfer on to a serving bowl. Sprinkle parsley. Drizzle olive oil on top and serve.

Israeli Eggplant Moussaka

Preparation time: 30 minutes

Cooking time: 45 minutes

Number of servings: 3

Ingredients:

- 1 tablespoon extra-virgin olive oil
- ½ pound ground turkey or lamb or beef or meatless crumbles
- 1/8 teaspoon ground cinnamon
- 1/8 teaspoon black pepper
- 1 can (14.5 ounces) tomato sauce
- ½ yellow onion, chopped
- ½ teaspoon minced garlic
- ¼ teaspoon salt
- 1 medium eggplant, cut into 1/3-inch-thick round slices
- ½ cup baba ganoush or hummus to serve

Directions:

1. Set the temperature of the oven to 400° F and preheat the oven.
2. Prepare a casserole dish by spraying it with nonstick cooking spray.

3. Pour oil into a heavy skillet and let it heat over medium heat. When oil is hot, add onion and cook until brown.
4. Stir in garlic and meat of choice and cook until brown. As you stir, break the meat into smaller pieces.
5. Stir in pepper, salt, and cinnamon and cook for a couple of minutes. Turn off the heat.
6. Spread half the eggplant slices on the bottom of the casserole dish. Spread half the meat mixture over the eggplant slices.
7. Spread half the tomato sauce over the meat mixture. Place remaining eggplant slices followed by remaining meat mixture and tomato sauce.
8. Keep the dish covered with aluminum foil. Place the baking dish in the oven and set the timer for 45 minutes.
9. Serve with hummus on top.

One Pan Za'atar Chicken and Rice

Preparation time: 20 minutes

Cooking time: 60 – 80 minutes

Number of servings: 2

Ingredients:

- ½ onion, diced
- 2 tablespoons extra-virgin olive oil, divided
- 2 tablespoons za'atar
- Kosher salt to taste
- 1 ½ cups hot chicken broth
- 1 clove garlic, minced
- 1 ½ pounds chicken, skinless, cut into 4 pieces
- Juice of ½ lemon
- ¾ cup uncooked basmati rice
- Toasted almonds to garnish
- Chopped parsley to garnish

Directions:

1. Set the temperature of the oven to 400° F and preheat the oven.
2. Combine onion, 1-tablespoon oil, and garlic in a casserole dish. Place in the oven and let it cook for 15 minutes.

3. Place chicken in a bowl. Drizzle 1 tablespoon of oil over the chicken and toss well.
4. Sprinkle za'atar and salt to taste. Mix well. Drizzle lemon juice over the chicken and toss well.
5. Take out the casserole dish from the oven and stir the rice into the onion mixture. Add about ½ teaspoon of salt and stir until well combined.
6. Lay the chicken pieces over the rice. Drizzle hot broth all over the rice and surrounding the chicken.
7. Keep the casserole dish covered with aluminum foil. Keep the casserole dish back in the oven and set the timer for 50 - 60 minutes or until chicken is early cooked and very little broth remaining in the casserole.
8. Uncover and trickle some more oil over the rice and chicken if desired. Bake for some more time until the chicken is brown on top and the rice is cooked.
9. Lift the chicken from the dish and place on a plate. Take a fork and loosen the rice. Add almonds and some za'atar to taste. Mix gently with a fork.
10. Divide rice into 2 plates. Place 2 chicken pieces on top on each plate and serve.

Chapter Seven: Israeli Desserts

Sahlab

Preparation time: 5 minutes

Cooking time: 10 minutes

Number of servings: 2

Ingredients:

- 2 cups milk of your choice
- 2 tablespoons sugar
- 4 drops vanilla extract
- 2 tablespoons cornstarch
- ½ teaspoon rose water

For topping:

- 2 teaspoons shelled pistachios
- Ground cinnamon to garnish
- 2 teaspoons desiccated coconut
- 2 teaspoons flaked or chopped almonds

Directions:

1. Pour 1 ½ cups milk into a saucepan and place the saucepan over medium-low heat.
2. Whisk together ½ cup milk, cornstarch, rose water, sugar, and vanilla in a bowl.

3. When the milk is very hot but not boiling, pour the milk mixture into the saucepan. Stir constantly until it starts boiling.
4. Continue stirring for a couple of minutes until thick.
5. Pour into 2 cups.
6. Sprinkle coconut, almonds, and pistachios on top. Finally garnish with cinnamon and serve.

Tahini Olive Oil Cake

Preparation time: 15 minutes

Cooking time: 30 minutes

Number of servings: 20 – 25

Ingredients:

- 1 cup extra-virgin olive oil
- 1 cup sugar
- 4 tablespoons lemon juice
- 1 cup honey
- 1 cup Sabra classic tahini
- 4 tablespoons grated lemon zest
- 3 cups all-purpose flour
- ½ teaspoon salt
- 1 teaspoon baking soda
- 2 teaspoons baking powder
- ½ teaspoon ground nutmeg
- 2 teaspoons ground cinnamon
- 1 teaspoon ground cardamom

To serve:

- Whipped cream
- Honey
- Grated lemon zest

- Fresh raspberries

Directions:

1. Set the temperature of the oven to 350° F and preheat the oven.
2. Prepare a large, round baking dish (9 – 10 inches) by greasing it with some cooking oil spray and place a sheet of parchment paper inside the baking dish. Spray the parchment paper too.
3. Place honey, sugar, and oil in the mixing bowl of the stand mixer. Beat until very smooth.
4. Beat in the tahini, lemon zest, and lemon juice.
5. Add flour, salt, spices, and baking soda into another bowl and stir until well combined.
6. Add the flour mixture into the mixing bowl and beat until just incorporated.
7. Transfer the batter into the prepared baking dish.
8. Place the baking dish in the oven and set the timing for 30 to 35 minutes or until brown on top and the cake is set in the middle.
9. Remove the baking dish from the oven and cool completely. Cover the cake with a foil tent loosely until use.
10. Top with the suggested serving options. Cut into slices and serve.

Baklava

Preparation time: minutes

Cooking time: minutes

Number of servings: 20 – 25

Ingredients:

For Baklava:

- 2 pounds phyllo dough, thawed
- 3 cups butter, melted
- 4 cups finely chopped nuts (pistachios or almonds or walnuts or hazelnuts or use a mixture)

For the syrup:

- 4 cups sugar
- 4 cups water
- 2 teaspoons lemon juice
- ½ cup honey
- 1 stick cinnamon
- Ground pistachios, to garnish (optional but recommended)

Directions:

1. Take a large baking dish (9 x 13 inches) and place on your countertop.
2. Unroll the dough and cut the sheets if desired to fit into the baking dish. Cover with a moist towel. This is necessary, as the sheets tend to dry.
3. Pull out a sheet of dough and place on the bottom of the baking dish. Cut the sheet to fit in if necessary.
4. Brush with butter. Place one more sheet over this.
5. Repeat the layers (previous step until you have 8 - 10 layers in all).
6. Spread a thin layer of the chopped nuts, all over the last layer after brushing the last layer with butter.
7. Place 2 phyllo sheets over the nut layer, brushing butter on each layer.
8. Repeat steps 6 – 7 until all the nut mixture is used up.
9. Now place remaining phyllo sheets over this, brushing each layer with butter. The topmost layer should also be brushed with butter. Cut into diamond shaped pieces.
10. Set the temperature of the oven to 350° F and preheat the oven. Place the baking dish in the oven and set the timer for 50 – 60 minutes or until light - medium golden brown on top and light brown and crisp on the edges.
11. Meanwhile prepare the syrup: Add water into a saucepan. Place the saucepan on medium heat. Add sugar, honey, cinnamon, and lemon juice and bring to a boil, lower heat

and simmer for 5-6 minutes. Stir frequently until sugar melts.

12. Lower the heat and simmer until slightly thick. Turn off the heat and cool completely. Remove from the oven.
13. Discard cinnamon sticks from the cooled syrup. Pour the syrup all over the top layer. The baked baklava should be hot when you pour the syrup.
14. Let the baklava cool completely.
15. Sprinkle pistachio nuts on top and serve.

Israeli Halvah

Preparation time: 5 minutes + stirring time + chilling time

Cooking time: 8 - 10 minutes

Number of servings: 10 – 12

Ingredients:

- ¾ cup tahini
- 1 cup honey
- ½ - 1 cup toasted, sliced almonds or nuts of your choice (optional)

Directions:

1. Pour honey into a saucepan. Place the saucepan over medium heat and heat the honey until the temperature of the honey shows 240° F on an instant-read thermometer.
2. Meanwhile, place tahini in a small pot and stir a few times. Place the pot over medium heat and heat tahini until the temperature shows 120° F on the instant read thermometer.
3. Now combine honey and tahini using a wooden spoon. Keep stirring for a few minutes until very smooth.
4. Stir in the nuts. Keep stirring for about 6 – 8 minutes and the mixture will start hardening.
5. Grease a loaf pan or springform pan with some butter or oil. Spoon the mixture into the pan.

6. Allow it to cool completely. Keep the loaf pan covered with cling wrap. Place in the refrigerator for 24 – 36 hours. Sugar crystals may be visible but that's perfectly ok, in fact it is great.
7. Invert the pan on your cutting board. Cut into slices.
8. Serve. The leftover slices should be wrapped tightly with cling wrap and placed in an airtight container in the refrigerator. It can last for 4 – 5 months.

Chocolate Rugelach

Preparation time: 40 minutes + resting time

Cooking time: 20 minutes

Number of servings: 15

Ingredients:

<u>For dough:</u>

- ¼ cup – 1/8 cup warm water 100° F
- 3 tablespoons caster sugar
- 3 tablespoons canola oil
- 8.8 – 9.7 ounces all-purpose flour
- ½ teaspoon ground cinnamon
- ¾ teaspoon instant dry yeast
- ¼ teaspoon salt
- 1 egg, at room temperature

<u>For chocolate filling:</u>

- 2 ½ tablespoons cocoa powder, unsweetened
- ¼ tablespoon ground cinnamon
- 3 tablespoons caster sugar
- 1 ½ tablespoons canola oil

<u>For egg wash:</u>

- ½ tablespoon water
- 1 small egg yolk

<u>For sugar syrup glaze:</u>

- 1 ½ tablespoons water
- 4 teaspoons caster sugar

Directions:

1. Combine warm water, ½ tablespoon sugar, and yeast in a bowl. Set it aside for a few minutes. In 5 – 10 minutes the solution will be a little frothy.
2. Add oil and egg and whisk until egg is mixed well.
3. Combine flour, cinnamon, and remaining sugar in the mixing bowl of the stand mixer. You can make the dough by using your hands as well.
4. Make a cavity in the center of the flour mixture and pour the yeast solution in the cavity. I am making the dough in the stand mixer. Fix the dough hook attachment and knead the dough for about 2 minutes. Sprinkle salt over the dough and continue kneading for about 10 minutes until you get soft and supple dough.
5. Grease a bowl generously with oil and place the dough in the bowl. Turn the dough around in the bowl to grease the dough.
6. Cover the bowl with a kitchen towel and place it in a warm area for a couple of hours or until it doubles in size.

7. To make chocolate filling: Add cocoa, water, sugar, and cinnamon into a bowl and stir until sugar dissolves completely.
8. Once the dough is ready, punch the dough. Divide the mixture into 2 equal portions and shape into balls.
9. Set the temperature of the oven to 350° F and preheat the oven. Prepare a baking sheet by lining it with parchment paper.
10. Dust your countertop with some flour. Place a ball of dough and roll into a round shape of around 1/8 inch thickness.
11. Spread some chocolate mixture over the dough, leaving the edges. Cut into wedges with a pizza cutter. The width of the wedge should be 1 – 1 ½ inches.
12. Separate the wedges from each other. Roll each wedge, from the wide side towards the thinner side, finally to the tip of the wedge.
13. Place on the baking sheet, with the seam side facing down.
14. For egg wash: Beat yolk and water in a bowl and whisk well.
15. Brush the top of the rolls with egg wash
16. Repeat the same process with another ball of dough.
17. Place the baking sheet in the oven and bake for about 30 minutes or until golden brown on top.
18. Meanwhile, make the sugar syrup glaze: Combine sugar and water in a saucepan and place the saucepan over medium-low heat. Let it simmer until you get thick syrup. Turn off the heat.

19. Remove from the oven and immediately brush the sugar syrup glaze over the rugelach. Cool completely. Store in an airtight container.

Honey Cake

Preparation time: 15 minutes

Cooking time: 50 – 60 minutes

Number of servings: 15 – 18

Ingredients:

- ½ teaspoon ground cinnamon
- ½ tablespoon baking powder
- ½ teaspoon baking soda
- 1 ¾ cups unbleached flour
- 2 tablespoons canola oil
- 2 extra-large eggs
- ¼ teaspoon ground ginger
- 1/8 teaspoon ground nutmeg
- ½ cup raisins
- ½ cup + 1/8 cup dark brown sugar
- ¾ cup + 1/8 cup honey
- ½ cup very strong coffee
- 1/8 teaspoon ground cloves
- ½ cup whole almonds

Directions:

1. Set the temperature of the oven to 300° F and preheat the oven. Prepare a baking dish (9 x 5 inches) by greasing it

with some cooking spray. Dust with some flour into the dish as well.

2. Add coffee and honey into a saucepan. Place the saucepan over medium heat. Stir occasionally.
3. When the mixture comes to a boil, turn off the heat and let it cool completely.
4. Meanwhile, sift together flour, baking soda, baking powder, ginger, nutmeg, cloves, and cinnamon in a bowl.
5. Crack eggs into a bowl. Add oil and brown sugar and whisk until well combined, making sure not to overbeat.
6. Add a little of the flour mixture into the bowl. Also add a little of the coffee mixture and stir until just combined.
7. Repeat this process (of adding flour mixture and coffee mixture) until all of it is added but the coffee mixture should be added finally.
8. Add raisins and stir. Spoon the batter into the baking dish.
9. Place almonds at equal distance all over the batter in such a manner that when you cut squares of the cake, there should be an almond in the center of the square.
10. Place the baking dish in the oven and set the timer for 60 – 70 minutes or until cooked through inside. To check this, insert a toothpick in the center of the cake and remove it. Check if there are any particles stuck on it. If it is stuck, then you have to bake for another 5 – 10 minutes, else turn off the oven and remove the baking dish.
11. Let it cool completely. Cover the cake and let it rest for 9 – 10 hours. Cut into squares and serve.
12. Store leftover cake in an airtight container.

Sweet Lokshen Kugel

Preparation time: 15 minutes

Cooking time: 50 – 60 minutes

Number of servings: 7 – 8

Ingredients:

- ½ cup raisins or craisins or dried chopped apricots or canned, drained, chopped pineapple
- 3 large eggs
- 4 ounces cottage cheese
- 1/8 cup butter, melted
- ½ teaspoon ground cinnamon to sprinkle
- 6 ounces wide egg noodles
- 1 cup sour cream
- ½ cup sugar + extra to sprinkle
- 1/8 teaspoon salt
- 4 ounces cream cheese

Directions:

1. Keep the rack in the center of the oven. Set the temperature of the oven to 350° F and preheat the oven. Grease a baking dish (about 6 x 6 inches) with cooking spray. Soak raisins or craisins or apricots in a bowl of hot water until the noodles are cooked, about 20 minutes.

2. Place a pot of water over high heat. When water starts boiling, add noodles. Cook until just al dente, making sure not to overcook. Turn off the heat.
3. Drain the noodles and add it back into the pot.
4. Place eggs, cottage cheese, sour cream, cream cheese, salt, butter, and sugar in a blender and blend until smooth.
5. Pour the blended mixture into the pot with noodles and mix well. Add raisins into the pot, after draining. Transfer the contents of the pot into the prepared baking dish. Give a sprinkle of cinnamon and a generous amount of sugar on top.
6. Place the baking dish in the oven and bake for 50 – 60 minutes or until golden brown on top. Take out the baking dish from the oven and let it rest for at least 15 minutes.
7. Cut into square pieces. This dish is to be served either cold or warm.

Apricot Hamantaschen

Preparation time: 20 minutes + chilling time

Cooking time: 15 minutes

Number of servings: 10

Ingredients:

- 1/3 cup confectioner's sugar
- ¼ teaspoon salt
- Yolk of a large egg, beaten
- ¼ cup apricot jam
- ¾ cup all-purpose flour + extra to dust
- 2.7 ounces chilled unsalted butter, cut into cubes
- 1 – 2 teaspoons ice water
- Yolk of a small egg for egg wash

Directions:

1. Place flour, confectioner's sugar, and salt in the food processor bowl and blend until well combined.
2. Scatter butter over the mixture and pulse until the mixture has a sand-like texture.
3. Add the large egg yolk and pulse until well combined. Pour about ½ tablespoon water into the mixture and pulse until the mixture starts to get sticky. If it doesn't, add another ½ tablespoon of water and pulse dough together.

4. Dust your countertop with a little flour. Place the dough on the countertop, over the dusted area and knead the dough with your hands until smooth dough is formed.
5. Flatten the dough ball and wrap it in cling wrap. Place it in the refrigerator for about 30 minutes.
6. Prepare a baking sheet by lining it with parchment paper.
7. Once again dust your countertop with some flour.
8. Take out the dough from the refrigerator and unwrap it. Place the dough on the dusted area.
9. Roll the dough until it is 1/8 inch thick. Keep dusting with more flour when necessary. Keep turning the dough while rolling.
10. Cut into cookies using a cookie cutter. Place the cut cookies on the baking sheet.
11. Now gather the scrap dough and re-roll into a ball of dough. Repeat steps 7 – 10 a couple of times and cut into cookies.
12. Brush egg wash lightly on the rolled dough. Take a spoonful of apricot jam and place it on the center of each of the cookies. Fold a little of the sides of the dough over the cookies and make the shape of a triangle. The jam should be visible in the center of the cookie so fold only a little of the edges of the rolled dough. Press the tips of the triangle so that they stick together.
13. Place the baking sheet in the refrigerator for about 20 minutes.
14. Set the temperature of the oven to 375° F and preheat the oven.

15. Place the baking sheet in the oven and bake for 12 – 15 minutes or until the edges and top start turning light golden brown.
16. Take out the baking sheet and let them cool for 5 – 8 minutes on the baking sheet itself.
17. Remove the cookies and place them on a wire rack for cooling.
18. Serve. Store leftovers in an airtight container.

Mandelbrot (Mandel Bread)

Preparation time: 15 minutes

Cooking time: 40 minutes

Number of servings: 12 – 14

Ingredients:

- 1/3 cup vegetable oil
- 1 large egg
- 1 cup all-purpose flour
- 1/8 teaspoon salt
- Ground cinnamon to dust
- Granulated sugar to dust
- 1/3 cup sugar
- 1/3 teaspoon pure vanilla extract
- 1/3 teaspoon baking powder
- 1/3 cup semi-sweet chocolate chips

Directions:

1. Add sugar and oil into the mixing bowl of the stand mixer and whisk until sugar dissolves.
2. Add egg and beat well. Now fix the dough hook attachment.
3. Sift together flour, baking powder, and salt into a bowl.

4. Add the flour mixture into the bowl of egg mixture, a little at a time and mix well each time.
5. You will have sticky dough. Add chocolate chips and stir until they are well distributed.
6. Keep the bowl covered with cling wrap and chill for 2 – 9 hours.
7. Set the temperature of the oven to 350° F and preheat the oven.
8. Form the dough into 2 equal rectangles of about 1-inch height and about 3 – 4 inches width.
9. Place the loaves on a baking sheet leaving sufficient gap between them. Set the timer for 25 minutes.
10. Take out the baking sheet from the oven and let it cool for a few minutes.
11. Now reduce the temperature of the oven to 250° F.
12. Cut the mandel bread into about 1 inch thick slices.
13. Combine ground cinnamon and sugar on a plate. Dredge the mandel bread slices in cinnamon sugar. Place them on the baking sheet, flat.
14. Place the baking sheet back in the oven and bake for 15 minutes or longer, until the way you prefer it cooked.
15. Let them cool completely. Transfer them into an airtight container.

Hanukkah Jelly Donut Recipe (Sufganiyah)

Preparation time: 40 minutes + rising time

Cooking time: 30 minutes

Number of servings: 6 – 7

Ingredients:

- 6 ounces lukewarm water
- 1 1/8 teaspoons instant yeast
- 2 tablespoons neutral-flavored vegetable oil
- 2 teaspoons vanilla extract
- ½ cup strained strawberry jam
- ¼ cup powdered sugar, to dust
- 2 tablespoons granulated sugar
- 1 ½ cups + 1/3 cup all-purpose flour + extra for dusting
- 1 large egg, at room temperature
- ½ teaspoon salt
- Oil to fry, as required

Directions:

1. Fix the dough hook attachment to the stand mixer.
2. Add water, flour, oil, vanilla, egg, salt, sugar, and yeast into the mixing bowl of the stand mixer.
3. Set the speed on low and mix for about 8 – 10 minutes or until sticky dough is formed.

4. Grease a bowl with a generous amount of oil. Place the dough in the bowl and turn it around in the bowl.

5. Keep the bowl covered with cling wrap and finally a tea towel. Place the bowl in a warm area for a couple of hours or until it doubles in size.

6. Dust your countertop with some flour.

7. Place the dough on the dusted area.

8. Roll the dough until it is ½ inch thick.

9. Cut into cookies using a 2-½ inch cookie cutter. Place the cut donuts on the baking sheet.

10. Now gather the scrap dough and re-roll into a ball of dough. Repeat steps 7 – 10 a couple of times and cut into cookies.

11. Dust the top of the donuts with some flour and keep the baking sheet covered with a tea towel.

12. Pour enough oil into a deep frying pan such that the oil is about 2 ½ - 3 inches in height from the bottom of the pan. Place the pan over medium heat and let the oil heat to 325° F.

13. Take another baking sheet and line it with paper towels. Place a wire rack on the baking sheet and keep this set up near your stovetop.

14. When the oil is hot and reaches 325° F, carefully lift a donut at a time and slide it into the oil. Fry 2 – 3 at a time. Turn occasionally and fry until golden brown. Remove the donuts with a slotted spoon and place on the rack.

15. Fry the remaining donuts in a similar manner.

16. Once they are cooled, take a skewer and pierce a hole on top of each donut, making sure the base of the donut is intact.
17. Fit a piping bag with a small, plain nozzle. Pour the jam into a piping bag and pipe the jam into the holes.
18. Sprinkle powdered sugar around the donuts.
19. Serve. You can store the leftover donuts in an airtight container. You can leave the container at room temperature. Use it within 2 days.

Tahini & Almond Cookies

Preparation time: 15 minutes

Cooking time: 15 minutes

Number of servings: 18

Ingredients:

- ½ cup all-purpose flour
- 1 cup ground almonds
- A pinch salt
- ½ cup tahini
- ½ teaspoon vanilla extract
- ½ cup whole-wheat flour
- 5 ½ tablespoons caster sugar
- 7 tablespoons unsalted butter, softened to room temperature
- 1 tablespoon water

Directions:

1. Set the temperature of the oven to 350° F and preheat the oven. Prepare a baking sheet by lining it with parchment paper.
2. Add flours, ground almonds, salt, sugar, and butter into the food processor bowl. Process until well combined and crumbly in texture.

3. Mix in water, tahini, and vanilla. Keep mixing until smooth dough is formed.

4. Dust your countertop with a little flour. Place the dough on the dusted area and knead until smooth.

5. Using a small ice cream scoop, scoop out the dough and place on the baking sheet. Leave sufficient gaps between the cookies. Press slightly with the back of a glass.

6. Place the baking sheet in the oven and bake until light golden brown in color, about 12 – 15 minutes.

7. Let the cookies remain on the baking sheet for about 5 – 8 minutes.

8. Loosen the cookies with a spatula and place on a wire rack. Let it cool completely.

9. Transfer into an airtight container.

Kanafeh

Preparation time: 20 minutes

Cooking time: 25 minutes

Number of servings: 4

Ingredients:

- 4 ounces kadaif angel hair
- 1/3 cup ghee also called clarified butter
- 1/8 teaspoon orange food coloring
- 8 ounces akkawi cheese
- 1.5 ounces crushed pistachios

<u>For syrup:</u>

- ¾ cup caster sugar
- ¼ cup water
- 1 ½ teaspoons rose water

Directions:

1. The previous day before preparing this dish, place akkawi cheese on your cutting board and cut into slices that are neither thick nor thin.
2. Place the slices in a large bowl of water. Drain and pour fresh water every 2 – 3 hours. Drain off the water finally.

3. Melt ghee in a small pan over low heat. Add food coloring and stir.
4. Add a little of the kadaif in a blender and give short pulses until they are smaller in size.
5. Remove into a bowl.
6. Repeat with the remaining kadaif. Add melted ghee and mix well using your hands.
7. Take a small baking dish and place more than half the kadaif on the bottom of the baking dish. Press the kadaif with your hands.
8. Now grate the cheese directly over the kadaif in the baking dish. Make sure the entire kadaif is covered with cheese.
9. Set the temperature of the oven to 350° F and preheat the oven. Place the baking dish in the oven.
10. To make syrup: Pour water into a saucepan. Add sugar and place the saucepan over medium-high heat.
11. When it comes to a boil, lower the heat to medium heat. Stir until sugar dissolves completely. Turn off the heat and add rose water. Mix well and keep it aside to cool completely.
12. Pour syrup over kanafeh. Scatter pistachios on top and serve.

Conclusion

According to the co-author of the book *'Zahav: A World of Israeli Cooking,'* Michael Solomonov, Israeli cuisine is a mix of many cuisines and cultures from around the world. These cuisines and cultures may have been in Israel for over a thousand years. It is impossible to summarize the list of foods included in Israeli cuisine, and a typical meal in an Israeli home may consist of at least 12 plates. Each of these foods has its roots in different cultures and countries. These dishes have a mix of different vegetables, grilled meats, tahini sauces and spices.

Israeli cuisine is not defined in definite terms, but it is a blend of different cuisines and cultures with over a thousand years of heritage. Israelis are still working with different foods and experimenting to create new dishes. This means the cuisine is still evolving. This book has delicious recipes with traditional ingredients. You can tweak these recipes to suit your tastes and make your version of Israeli foods. This book has recipes for some of the most famous Israeli foods.

If you cannot find some ingredients listed in the recipe, swap it with one of your own. You can look for substitutes if you want to, as well. I hope you and your family enjoy the recipes in the book.

Resources

https://www.jpost.com/israel-news/culture/israeli-cuisine-how-did-we-get-here-512040

https://www.myjewishlearning.com/article/israeli-food-after-1948/

https://www.myjewishlearning.com/article/israeli-food/

https://www.10best.com/interests/food-culture/the-essential-ingredients-that-define-israeli-cuisine/

https://www.touristisrael.com/israel-best-foods/28233/

The end... almost!

Reviews are not easy to come by.

As an independent author with a tiny marketing budget, I rely on readers, like you, to leave a short review on Amazon.

Even if it's just a sentence or two!

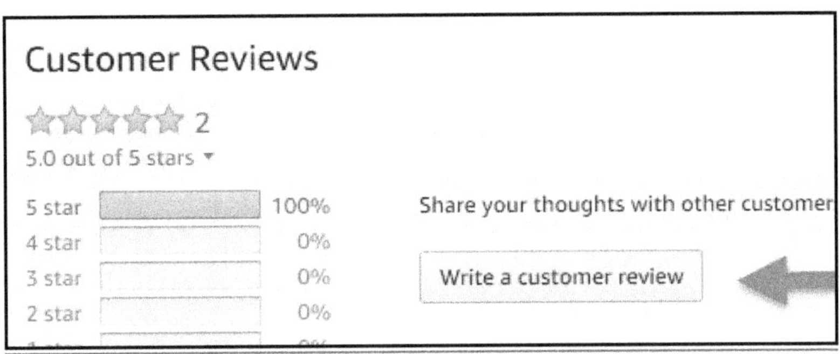

So if you enjoyed the book, please...

I am very appreciative for your review as it truly makes a difference.

Thank you from the bottom of my heart for purchasing this book and reading it to the end.